BLACKWELL'S
UNDERGROUND CLINICAL VIGNETTES

SURGERY, 2E

BLACKWELL'S
UNDERGROUND CLINICAL VIGNETTES

SURGERY, 2E

VIKAS BHUSHAN, MD
University of California, San Francisco, Class of 1991
Series Editor, Diagnostic Radiologist

VISHAL PALL, MBBS
Government Medical College, Chandigarh, India, Class of 1996
Series Editor, U. of Texas, Galveston, Resident in Internal Medicine &
Preventive Medicine

TAO LE, MD
University of California, San Francisco, Class of 1996

FADI ABOU-NUKTA, MD
University of Damascus, Syria, Class of 1998

YI-MENG YEN, MD, PHD
University of California, Los Angeles, Resident in Orthopaedic Surgery

VIPAL SONI, MD
UCLA School of Medicine, Class of 1999

Blackwell
Science

CONTRIBUTORS

Mimi Kim, MD
Indiana University School of Medicine, Indianapolis,
Resident in Surgery

Hoang Nguyen, MD, MBA
Northwestern University, Class of 2001

John Schilling, MD
University of Chicago, Class of 1999

Linh Nguyen, MD
University of Illinois, Chicago, Resident in Surgery

Jose Fierro, MBBS
La Salle University, Mexico City

© 2002 by Blackwell Science, Inc.

Editorial Offices:
Commerce Place, 350 Main Street, Malden,
   Massachusetts 02148, USA
Osney Mead, Oxford OX2 0EL, England
25 John Street, London WC1N 2BS, England
23 Ainslie Place, Edinburgh EH3 6AJ, Scotland
54 University Street, Carlton, Victoria 3053,
   Australia

Other Editorial Offices:
Blackwell Wissenschafts-Verlag GmbH,
   Kurfürstendamm 57, 10707 Berlin, Germany
Blackwell Science KK, MG Kodenmacho Building,
   7-10 Kodenmacho Nihombashi, Chuo-ku,
   Tokyo 104, Japan
Iowa State University Press, A Blackwell Science
   Company, 2121 S. State Avenue, Ames, Iowa
   50014-8300, USA

Distributors:
The Americas
Blackwell Publishing
c/o AIDC
P.O. Box 20
50 Winter Sport Lane
Williston, VT 05495-0020
(Telephone orders: 800-216-2522;
   fax orders: 802-864-7626)
Australia
Blackwell Science Pty, Ltd.
54 University Street
Carlton, Victoria 3053
(Telephone orders: 03-9347-0300;
   fax orders: 03-9349-3016)
Outside The Americas and Australia
Blackwell Science, Ltd.
c/o Marston Book Services, Ltd.
P.O. Box 269
Abingdon
Oxon OX14 4YN
England
(Telephone orders: 44-01235-465500;
   fax orders: 44-01235-465555)

Acquisitions: Laura DeYoung
Development: Amy Nuttbrock
Production: Lorna Hind and Shawn Girsberger
Manufacturing: Lisa Flanagan
Marketing Manager: Kathleen Mulcahy
Cover design by Leslie Haimes
Interior design by Shawn Girsberger
Typeset by TechBooks
Printed and bound by Capital City Press

Blackwell's Underground Clinical Vignettes:
   Surgery, 2e
ISBN 0-632-04575-2

Printed in the United States of America
02 03 04 05 5 4 3 2 1

The Blackwell Science logo is a trade mark of
Blackwell Science Ltd., registered at the United
Kingdom Trade Marks Registry

Library of Congress Cataloging-in-Publication Data
Bhushan, Vikas.
Blackwell's underground clinical vignettes.
Surgery / author, Vikas Bhushan. – 2nd ed.
    p. ; cm. – (Underground clinical vignettes) Rev. ed.
of: Surgery / Vikas Bhushan ... [et al.].
c1999. ISBN 0-632-04575-2 (pbk.)
1. Surgery – Case studies. 2. Physicians – Licenses –
United States – Examinations – Study guides.
    [DNLM: 1. Surgical Procedures, Operative –
Case Report. 2. Surgical Procedures, Operative –
Problems and Exercises. WO 18.2 B575b 2002]
I. Title: Underground clinical vignettes. Surgery.
II. Title: Surgery. III. Surgery. IV. Title. V. Series.
   RD34 .B48 2002
   617–dc21

                                    2001004888

CONTENTS

MINICASES

ACKNOWLEDGMENTS

Throughout the production of this book, we have had the support of many friends and colleagues. Special thanks to our support team including Anu Gupta, Andrea Fellows, Anastasia Anderson, Srishti Gupta, Mona Pall, Jonathan Kirsch and Chirag Amin. For prior contributions we thank Gianni Le Nguyen, Tarun Mathur, Alex Grimm, Sonia Santos and Elizabeth Sanders.

We have enjoyed working with a world-class international publishing group at Blackwell Science, including Laura DeYoung, Amy Nuttbrock, Lisa Flanagan, Shawn Girsberger, Lorna Hind and Gordon Tibbitts. For help with securing images for the entire series we also thank Lee Martin, Kristopher Jones, Tina Panizzi and Peter Anderson at the University of Alabama, the Armed Forces Institute of Pathology, and many of our fellow Blackwell Science authors.

For submitting comments, corrections, editing, proofreading, and assistance across all of the vignette titles in all editions, we collectively thank:

Tara Adamovich, Carolyn Alexander, Kris Alden, Henry E. Aryan, Lynman Bacolor, Natalie Barteneva, Dean Bartholomew, Debashish Behera, Sumit Bhatia, Sanjay Bindra, Dave Brinton, Julianne Brown, Alexander Brownie, Tamara Callahan, David Canes, Bryan Casey, Aaron Caughey, Hebert Chen, Jonathan Cheng, Arnold Cheung, Arnold Chin, Simion Chiosea, Yoon Cho, Samuel Chung, Gretchen Conant, Vladimir Coric, Christopher Cosgrove, Ronald Cowan, Karekin R. Cunningham, A. Sean Dalley, Rama Dandamudi, Sunit Das, Ryan Armando Dave, John David, Emmanuel de la Cruz, Robert DeMello, Navneet Dhillon, Sharmila Dissanaike, David Donson, Adolf Etchegaray, Alea Eusebio, Priscilla A. Frase, David Frenz, Kristin Gaumer, Yohannes Gebreegziabher, Anil Gehi, Tony George, L.M. Gotanco, Parul Goyal, Alex Grimm, Rajeev Gupta, Ahmad Halim, Sue Hall, David Hasselbacher, Tamra Heimert, Michelle Higley, Dan Hoit, Eric Jackson, Tim Jackson, Sundar Jayaraman, Pei-Ni Jone, Aarchan Joshi, Rajni K. Jutla, Faiyaz Kapadi, Seth Karp, Aaron S. Kesselheim, Sana Khan, Andrew Pin-wei Ko, Francis Kong, Paul Konitzky, Warren S. Krackov, Benjamin H.S. Lau, Ann LaCasce, Connie Lee, Scott Lee, Guillermo Lehmann, Kevin Leung, Paul Levett, Warren Levinson, Eric Ley, Ken Lin,

Pavel Lobanov, J. Mark Maddox, Aram Mardian, Samir Mehta, Gil Melmed, Joe Messina, Robert Mosca, Michael Murphy, Vivek Nandkarni, Siva Naraynan, Carvell Nguyen, Linh Nguyen, Deanna Nobleza, Craig Nodurft, George Noumi, Darin T. Okuda, Adam L. Palance, Paul Pamphrus, Jinha Park, Sonny Patel, Ricardo Pietrobon, Riva L. Rahl, Aashita Randeria, Rachan Reddy, Beatriu Reig, Marilou Reyes, Jeremy Richmon, Tai Roe, Rick Roller, Rajiv Roy, Diego Ruiz, Anthony Russell, Sanjay Sahgal, Urmimala Sarkar, John Schilling, Isabell Schmitt, Daren Schuhmacher, Sonal Shah, Edie Shen, Justin Smith, John Stulak, Lillian Su, Julie Sundaram, Rita Suri, Seth Sweetser, Antonio Talayero, Merita Tan, Mark Tanaka, Eric Taylor, Jess Thompson, Indi Trehan, Raymond Turner, Okafo Uchenna, Eric Uyguanco, Richa Varma, John Wages, Alan Wang, Eunice Wang, Andy Weiss, Amy Williams, Brian Yang, Hany Zaky, Ashraf Zaman and David Zipf.

For generously contributing images to the entire *Underground Clinical Vignette* Step 2 series, we collectively thank the staff at Blackwell Science in Oxford, Boston, and Berlin as well as:

- Alfred Cuschieri, Thomas P.J. Hennessy, Roger M. Greenhalgh, David I. Rowley, Pierce A. Grace (*Clinical Surgery*, © 1996 Blackwell Science), Figures 13.23, 13.35b, 13.51, 15.13, 15.2.

- John Axford (*Medicine*, © 1996 Blackwell Science), Figures f3.10, 2.103a, 2.110b, 3.20a, 3.20b, 3.25b, 3.38a, 5.9Bi, 5.9Bii, 6.41a, 6.41b, 6.74b, 6.74c, 7.78ai, 7.78aii, 7.78b, 8.47b, 9.9e, f3.17, f3.36, f3.37, f5.27, f5.28, f5.45a, f5.48, f5.49a, f5.50, f5.65a, f5.67, f5.68, f8.27a, 10.120b, 11.63b, 11.63c, 11.68a, 11.68b, 11.68c, 12.37a, 12.37b.

- Peter Armstrong, Martin L. Wastie (*Diagnostic Imaging, 4ᵗʰ Edition*, © 1998 Blackwell Science), Figures 2.100, 2.108d, 2.109, 2.11, 2.112, 2.121, 2.122, 2.13, 2.1ba, 2.1bb, 2.36, 2.53, 2.54, 2.69a, 2.71, 2.80a, 2.81b, 2.82, 2.84a, 2.84b, 2.88, 2.89a, 2.89b, 2.90b, 2.94a, 2.94b, 2.96, 2.97, 2.98a, 2.98c, 3.11, 3.19, 3.20, 3.21, 3.22, 3.28, 3.30, 3.34, 3.35b, 3.35c, 3.36, 4.7, 4.8, 4.9, 5.29, 5.33, 5.58, 5.62, 5.63, 5.64, 5.65b, 5.66a, 5.66b, 5.69, 5.71, 5.75, 5.8, 5.9, 6.17a, 6.17b, 6.25, 6.28, 6.29c, 6.30, 7.13, 7.17a, 7.45a, 7.45b, 7.46, 7.50, 7.52, 7.53a, 7.57a, 7.58, 8.7a, 8.7b, 8.7c, 8.86, 8.8a, 8.96, 8.9a, 9.17a, 9.17b, 10.13a, 10.13b, 10.14a, 10.14b, 10.14c, 10.17a, 10.17b, 11.16b, 11.17a, 11.17b, 11.19, 11.23, 11.24, 11.2b, 11.2d, 11.30a, 11.30b, 12.12, 12.15,

12.18, 12.19, 12.3, 12.4, 12.8a, 12.8b, 13.13a, 13.18, 13.18a, 13.20, 13.22a, 13.22b, 13.29, 14.14a, 14.5, 14.6a, 15.25b, 15.29b, 15.31, 15.37, 17.4.

- N.C. Hughes-Jones, S. N. Wickramasinghe (*Lecture Notes On: Haematology, 6th Edition*, © 1996 Blackwell Science), Figures 2.1b, 2.2a, 3.14, 3.8, 4.3, 5.2b, 5.5a, 5.8, 7.1, 7.2, 7.3, 7.5, 8.1, 10.5b, 10.6, 11.1, plate 29, plate 34, plate 44, plate 45, plate 48, plate 5, plate 42.

- Thomas Grumme, Wolfgang Kluge, Konrad Kretzschmar, Andreas Roesler (*Cerebral and Spinal Computed Tomography, 3rd Edition*, © 1998 Blackwell Science), Figures 16.2b, 16.3, 16.6a, 17.1a, 18-1c, 18-5, 41.3c, 41.3d, 44.3, 46.8, 47.7, 48.2, 48.6a, 53.5, 55.2a, 55.2c, 56.2b, 57.1, 61.3a, 61.3b, 63.1a, 64.3a, 65.3c, 66.3b, 67.6, 70.1a, 70.3, 81.2a, 81.4, 82.2, 82.3, 84.6.

- P.R. Patel (*Lecture Notes On: Radiology*, © 1998 Blackwell Science), Figures 2.15, 2.16, 2.25, 2.26, 2.30, 2.31, 2.33, 2.36, 3.11, 3.16, 3.19, 3.4, 3.7, 4.19, 4.20, 4.38, 4.44, 4.45, 4.46, 4.47, 4.49, 4.5, 5.14, 5.6, 6.18, 6.19, 6.20, 6.21, 6.22, 6.31a, 6.31b, 7.18, 7.19, 7.21, 7.22, 7.32, 7.34, 7.41, 7.46a, 7.46b, 7.48, 7.49, 7.9, 8.2, 8.3, 8.4, 8.5, 8.8, 8.9, 9.12, 9.2, 9.3, 9.8, 9.9, 10.11, 10.16, 10.5.

- Ramsay Vallance (*An Atlas of Diagnostic Radiology in Gastroenterology*, © 1999 Blackwell Science), Figures 1.22, 2.57, 2.27, 2.55a, 2.58, 2.59, 2.63, 2.64, 2.65, 3.11, 3.3, 3.37, 3.39, 3.4, 4.6a, 4.8, 4.9, 5.1, 5.29, 5.63, 5.64b, 5.65b, 5.66b, 5.68a, 5.68b, 6.110, 6.15, 6.17, 6.23, 6.29b, 6.30, 6.39, 6.64a, 6.64b, 6.75, 6.78, 6.80, 7.57a, 7.57c, 7.60a, 8.17, 8.48, 8.53, 8.66, 9.11a, 9.15, 9.17, 9.23, 9.24, 9.25, 9.28, 9.30, 9.32a, 9.33, 9.43, 9.45, 9.55b, 9.57, 9.63, 9.64a, 9.64b, 9.64c, 9.66, 10.28, 10.36, 10.44, 10.6.

Please let us know if your name has been missed or misspelled and we will be happy to make the update in the next edition.

PREFACE TO THE 2ND EDITION

We were very pleased with the overwhelmingly positive student feedback for the 1st edition of our *Underground Clinical Vignettes* series. Well over 100,000 copies of the UCV books are in print and have been used by students all over the world.

Over the last two years we have accumulated and incorporated **over a thousand "updates"** and improvements suggested by you, our readers, including:

- many additions of specific boards and wards testable content

- deletions of redundant and overlapping cases

- reordering and reorganization of all cases in both series

- a new master index by case name in each Atlas

- correction of a few factual errors

- diagnosis and treatment updates

- addition of 5–20 new cases in every book

- and the addition of clinical exam photographs within *UCV— Anatomy*

And most important of all, the second edition sets now include two brand new **COLOR ATLAS** supplements, one for each Clinical Vignette series.

- The *UCV–Basic Science Color Atlas* (*Step 1*) includes over 250 color plates, divided into gross pathology, microscopic pathology (histology), hematology, and microbiology (smears).

- The *UCV–Clinical Science Color Atlas* (*Step 2*) has over 125 color plates, including patient images, dermatology, and funduscopy.

Each atlas image is descriptively captioned and linked to its corresponding Step 1 case, Step 2 case, and/or Step 2 MiniCase.

How Atlas Links Work:

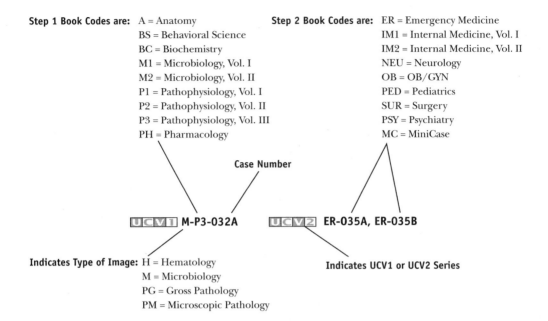

Step 1 Book Codes are:
A = Anatomy
BS = Behavioral Science
BC = Biochemistry
M1 = Microbiology, Vol. I
M2 = Microbiology, Vol. II
P1 = Pathophysiology, Vol. I
P2 = Pathophysiology, Vol. II
P3 = Pathophysiology, Vol. III
PH = Pharmacology

Step 2 Book Codes are:
ER = Emergency Medicine
IM1 = Internal Medicine, Vol. I
IM2 = Internal Medicine, Vol. II
NEU = Neurology
OB = OB/GYN
PED = Pediatrics
SUR = Surgery
PSY = Psychiatry
MC = MiniCase

Case Number

UCV1 M-P3-032A   UCV2 ER-035A, ER-035B

Indicates Type of Image:
H = Hematology
M = Microbiology
PG = Gross Pathology
PM = Microscopic Pathology

Indicates UCV1 or UCV2 Series

- If the Case number (032, 035, etc.) is not followed by a letter, then there is only one image. Otherwise A, B, C, D indicate up to 4 images.

Bold Faced Links: In order to give you access to the largest number of images possible, we have chosen to cross link the Step 1 and 2 series.

- If the link is bold-faced this indicates that the link is direct (i.e., Step 1 Case with the Basic Science Step 1 Atlas link).

- If the link is not bold-faced this indicates that the link is indirect (Step 1 case with Clinical Science Step 2 Atlas link or vice versa).

We have also implemented a few structural changes upon your request:

- Each current and future edition of our popular *First Aid for the USMLE Step 1* (Appleton & Lange/McGraw-Hill) and *First Aid for the USMLE Step 2* (Appleton & Lange/McGraw-Hill) book will be linked to the corresponding UCV case.

- We eliminated UCV → First Aid links as they frequently become out of date, as the *First Aid* books are revised yearly.

- The Color Atlas is also specially designed for quizzing—captions are descriptive and do not give away the case name directly.

New "MiniCases" replace the previous "Associated Diseases." There are now over **350 unique MiniCases** distributed throughout the ***Step 2 Clinical*** series, selected based on recent USMLE recollections.

We hope the updated UCV series will remain a unique and well-integrated study tool that provides compact clinical correlations to basic science information. They are designed to be easy and fun (comparatively) to read, and helpful for both licensing exams and the wards.

We invite your corrections and suggestions for the fourth edition of these books. For the first submission of each factual correction or new vignette that is selected for inclusion in the fourth edition, you will receive a personal acknowledgement in the revised book. If you submit over 20 high-quality corrections, additions or new vignettes we will also consider **inviting you to become a "Contributor" on the book of your choice**. If you are interested in becoming a potential "Contributor" or "Author" on a future UCV book, or working with our team in developing additional books, please also e-mail us your CV/resume.

We prefer that you submit corrections or suggestions via electronic mail to **UCVteam@yahoo.com**. Please include "Underground Vignettes" as the subject of your message. If you do not have access to e-mail, use the following mailing address: Blackwell Publishing, Attn: UCV Editors, 350 Main Street, Malden, MA 02148, USA.

Vikas Bhushan
Vishal Pall
Tao Le
October 2001

This series was originally developed to address the increasing number of clinical vignette questions on medical examinations, including the USMLE Step 1 and Step 2. It is also designed to supplement and complement the popular *First Aid for the USMLE Step 1* (Appleton & Lange/McGraw Hill) and *First Aid for the USMLE Step 2* (Appleton & Lange/McGraw Hill).

Each UCV 2 book uses a series of approximately 50 **"supra-prototypical" cases as a way to condense testable facts and associations**. The clinical vignettes in this series are designed to give added emphasis to pathogenesis, epidemiology, management and complications. They also contain relevant extensive B/W imaging plates within each book. Additionally, each UCV2 book contains approximately 30 to 60 "MiniCases" that focus on presenting only the key facts for that disease in a tightly edited fashion.

Although each case tends to present all the signs, symptoms, and diagnostic findings for a particular illness, **patients generally will not present with such a "complete" picture either clinically or on a medical examination**. Cases are not meant to simulate a potential real patient or an exam vignette. All the **boldfaced "buzzwords" are for learning purposes** and are not necessarily expected to be found in any one patient with the disease.

Definitions of selected important terms are placed within the vignettes in (SMALL CAPS) in parentheses. Other parenthetical remarks often refer to the pathophysiology or mechanism of disease. The format should also help students learn to present cases succinctly during oral "bullet" presentations on clinical rotations. The cases are meant to serve as a condensed review, not as a primary reference. The information provided in this book has been prepared with a great deal of thought and careful research. This book should not, however, be considered as your sole source of information. Corrections, suggestions and submissions of new cases are encouraged and will be acknowledged and incorporated when appropriate in future editions.

ABBREVIATIONS

5-ASA	5-aminosalicylic acid
ABGs	arterial blood gases
ABVD	adriamycin/bleomycin/vincristine/dacarbazine
ACE	angiotensin-converting enzyme
ACTH	adrenocorticotropic hormone
ADH	antidiuretic hormone
AFP	alpha fetal protein
AI	aortic insufficiency
AIDS	acquired immunodeficiency syndrome
ALL	acute lymphocytic leukemia
ALT	alanine transaminase
AML	acute myelogenous leukemia
ANA	antinuclear antibody
ARDS	adult respiratory distress syndrome
ASD	atrial septal defect
ASO	anti-streptolysin O
AST	aspartate transaminase
AV	arteriovenous
BE	barium enema
BP	blood pressure
BUN	blood urea nitrogen
CAD	coronary artery disease
CALLA	common acute lymphoblastic leukemia antigen
CBC	complete blood count
CHF	congestive heart failure
CK	creatine kinase
CLL	chronic lymphocytic leukemia
CML	chronic myelogenous leukemia
CMV	cytomegalovirus
CNS	central nervous system
COPD	chronic obstructive pulmonary disease
CPK	creatine phosphokinase
CSF	cerebrospinal fluid
CT	computed tomography
CVA	cerebrovascular accident
CXR	chest x-ray
DIC	disseminated intravascular coagulation
DIP	distal interphalangeal
DKA	diabetic ketoacidosis
DM	diabetes mellitus
DTRs	deep tendon reflexes
DVT	deep venous thrombosis

EBV	Epstein–Barr virus
ECG	electrocardiography
Echo	echocardiography
EF	ejection fraction
EGD	esophagogastroduodenoscopy
EMG	electromyography
ERCP	endoscopic retrograde cholangiopancreatography
ESR	erythrocyte sedimentation rate
FEV	forced expiratory volume
FNA	fine needle aspiration
FTA-ABS	fluorescent treponemal antibody absorption
FVC	forced vital capacity
GFR	glomerular filtration rate
GH	growth hormone
GI	gastrointestinal
GM-CSF	granulocyte macrophage colony stimulating factor
GU	genitourinary
HAV	hepatitis A virus
hcG	human chorionic gonadotrophin
HEENT	head, eyes, ears, nose, and throat
HIV	human immunodeficiency virus
HLA	human leukocyte antigen
HPI	history of present illness
HR	heart rate
HRIG	human rabies immune globulin
HS	hereditary spherocytosis
ID/CC	identification and chief complaint
IDDM	insulin-dependent diabetes mellitus
Ig	immunoglobulin
IGF	insulin-like growth factor
IM	intramuscular
JVP	jugular venous pressure
KUB	kidneys/ureter/bladder
LDH	lactate dehydrogenase
LES	lower esophageal sphincter
LFTs	liver function tests
LP	lumbar puncture
LV	left ventricular
LVH	left ventricular hypertrophy
Lytes	electrolytes
MCHC	mean corpuscular hemoglobin concentration
MCV	mean corpuscular volume
MEN	multiple endocrine neoplasia

MGUS	monoclonal gammopathy of undetermined significance
MHC	major histocompatibility complex
MI	myocardial infarction
MOPP	mechlorethamine/vincristine (Oncovorin)/procarbazine/prednisone
MR	magnetic resonance (imaging)
NHL	non-Hodgkin's lymphoma
NIDDM	non-insulin-dependent diabetes mellitus
NPO	nil per os (nothing by mouth)
NSAID	nonsteroidal anti-inflammatory drug
PA	posteroanterior
PIP	proximal interphalangeal
PBS	peripheral blood smear
PE	physical exam
PFTs	pulmonary function tests
PMI	point of maximal intensity
PMN	polymorphonuclear leukocyte
PT	prothrombin time
PTCA	percutaneous transluminal angioplasty
PTH	parathyroid hormone
PTT	partial thromboplastin time
PUD	peptic ulcer disease
RBC	red blood cell
RPR	rapid plasma reagin
RR	respiratory rate
RS	Reed–Sternberg (cell)
RV	right ventricular
RVH	right ventricular hypertrophy
SBFT	small bowel follow-through
SIADH	syndrome of inappropriate secretion of ADH
SLE	systemic lupus erythematosus
STD	sexually transmitted disease
TFTs	thyroid function tests
tPA	tissue plasminogen activator
TSH	thyroid-stimulating hormone
TIBC	total iron-binding capacity
TIPS	transjugular intrahepatic portosystemic shunt
TPO	thyroid peroxidase
TSH	thyroid-stimulating hormone
TTP	thrombotic thrombocytopenic purpura
UA	urinalysis
UGI	upper GI
US	ultrasound

VDRL	Venereal Disease Research Laboratory
VS	vital signs
VT	ventricular tachycardia
WBC	white blood cell
WPW	Wolff–Parkinson–White (syndrome)
XR	x-ray

ID/CC   A 31-year-old **woman** experiences progressively worsening **shortness of breath** while playing sports (EXERTIONAL DYSPNEA).

HPI   Over the past 6 months, she has become increasingly **fatigued** and has recently experienced recurring palpitations.

PE   VS: **tachycardia** (HR 120); hypotension (BP 90/60). PE: **no cyanosis**; prominent jugular venous v wave; **left parasternal heave** (RVH); midsystolic ejection murmur in pulmonic area; **widely split, fixed S$_2$** (from delayed pulmonic valve closure caused by increased volume in right ventricle); mid-diastolic rumble louder on inspiration (due to increased tricuspid flow); systolic flow murmur at lower left sternal border.

Labs   ECG: **atrial fibrillation** (due to atrial dilatation); right axis deviation; **RVH**; incomplete right bundle branch block.

Imaging   **[A]** CXR: **increased pulmonary vascularity** (due to left-to-right shunt); dilated pulmonary arteries; **right atrium and right ventricle enlarged**; small aortic knob (1) (due to diminished aortic blood flow). Echo: RA and RV enlargement; anterior systolic

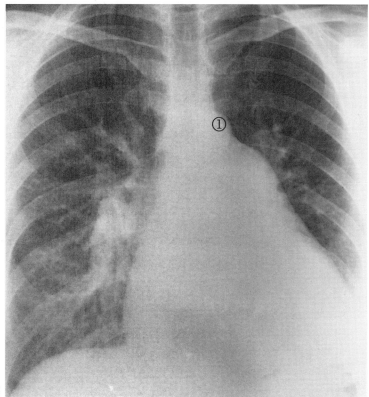

[A]

ATRIAL SEPTAL DEFECT

(PARADOXICAL) septal movement with transatrial blood flow. Angio: confirmatory; left-to-right atrial flow; O_2 saturation greater in right ventricle than in superior vena cava.

Pathogenesis Atrial septal defects (ASDs) are congenital left-to-right shunts. Three types exist. Approximately 80% of ASDs are **ostium secundum** defects involving the fossa ovalis. They are usually asymptomatic until adulthood, when pulmonary hypertension may develop, converting the left-to-right shunt to a right-to-left shunt (EISENMENGER'S SYNDROME). **Ostium primum** defects arise inferior to the fossa ovalis and are associated with **AV valve abnormalities** and **Down's syndrome**. These commonly present with **heart failure in childhood. Sinus venosus** defects arise high in the septum and are associated with anomalous pulmonary venous return.

Epidemiology More common in females (2:1); **accounts for 30% of congenital heart disease in adults**.

Management **Defect closure** via **surgical patching** or **invasive angiography**. Surgery is indicated for ostium secundum defects. Primum defects frequently require repair of mitral valve insufficiency, and sinus venosus defects may need a prosthesis. Contraindications to surgery include small, hemodynamically insignificant defects (ratio of pulmonary flow to systemic flow less than 1:2), longstanding pulmonary hypertension, and Eisenmenger's syndrome (may produce postoperative acute heart failure). **The ideal age for surgery is 3 to 6 years**.

Complications Paradoxic emboli, arrhythmias, heart failure (right-sided) and pulmonary hypertension (especially in primum defects).

Atlas Link ⬚Ｕ⬚Ｃ⬚Ｖ⬚Ｉ⬚ PG-A-002

ID/CC A 24-year-old **man** complains of recurrent **headaches** and **nosebleeds**.

HPI The patient occasionally experiences dizziness, cold extremities, claudication, palpitations, and dyspnea on exertion. He has a history of hypertension.

PE VS: **BP in arms 180/90** and in **legs 90/60**; no fever; normal RR. PE: no jaundice, pallor, or cyanosis; **harsh, late systolic ejection murmur heard in the interscapular area**; palpable pulsatile collaterals in intercostal spaces; **weak lower-extremity pulses**; neurologic and musculoskeletal exams normal.

Labs CBC: increased hematocrit. ECG: tall R in V_5 and V_6; deep S in V_1 and V_2; LVH.

Imaging CXR: enlarged aortic knob; **[A] rib notching** at the inferior margin of ribs 4 to 9 (collateral circulation). **[B]** Echo/MR/Angio: **indentation of the aorta at the level of coarctation with pre- and poststenotic dilatation** ("FIGURE OF THREE").

Pathogenesis The etiology of coarctation is unknown. Coarctation is usually **distal to the subclavian artery.** In the **infantile type,** it is

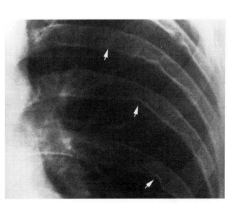

[A]

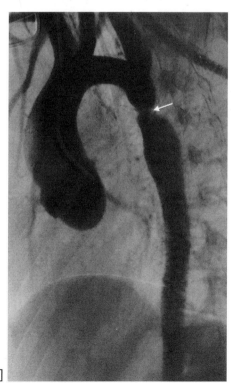

[B]

COARCTATION OF THE AORTA

proximal to the ligamentum arteriosum between the subclavian artery and the ductus arteriosus; infants with PDA may have equal upper-extremity and lower-extremity pulses. In the **adult type**, it is distal to the ligamentum arteriosum. The disease may range in severity from heart failure in infants to a lack of symptoms in adolescents and young adults, who are found to have hypertension on routine physicals. Symptomatic patients may complain of **headache**, weakness, **epistaxis**, fatigue, cold legs, intermittent claudication (calf pain while exercising), numbness of the legs, and **differential cyanosis** (unsaturated blood from right ventricle passes to the systemic circulation through the PDA).

Epidemiology
Coarctation of the aorta has a **male** predominance of 2 to 1 and is associated with **bicuspid aortic valve, Turner's syndrome**, VSD, endocardial cushion defect, mitral regurgitation, and PDA.

Management
Control of hypertension; prophylaxis against infectious endocarditis; surgical resection of the stenotic area with an end-to-end anastomosis or grafting, or invasive percutaneous balloon dilatation (BALLOON ANGIOPLASTY).

Complications
Most complications are secondary to hypertension and include cerebral aneurysms, bacterial endocarditis, aortic rupture, heart failure, and aortic dissection.

Atlas Link
UCV1 PG-A-004

ID/CC A 3-year-old boy presents with several **syncopal episodes** in which he **turned blue**.

HPI **Squatting relieves his symptoms** (increases peripheral vascular resistance, decreasing the right-to-left shunt). His parents also remark that he develops **blue nails and lips** while crying and straining.

PE VS: tachycardia. PE: small for age; **clubbing** of fingers and toes; **systolic thrill** at left sternal border (due to VSD); parasternal lift (due to RVH); **systolic ejection murmur** (due to pulmonary stenosis); murmur disappears during cyanotic spells (decreased blood flow through pulmonic valve); single S_2 (inaudible P_2 due to pulmonary stenosis).

Labs CBC: **elevated hemoglobin** (17.4 gm/dL) **and hematocrit** (66%); O_2 saturation 72%. ESR elevated. ECG: right axis deviation; RVH.

Imaging [A] CXR: small heart; rounded, upward-pointing apical shadow with concavity in the region of the main pulmonary artery

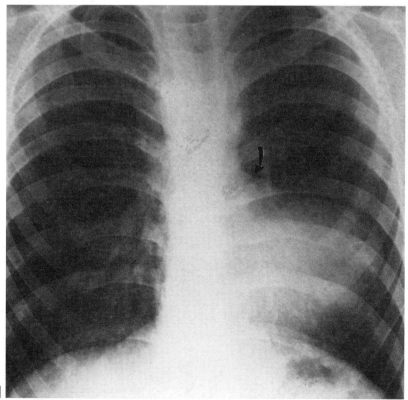

[A]

TETRALOGY OF FALLOT

(BOOT-SHAPED HEART); **diminished pulmonary vascularity** with unusually clear lung fields.

Pathogenesis The etiology of tetralogy of Fallot is unknown; cyanosis results from right-to-left shunting of blood across the VSD. Four defects are involved: large **VSD; RV outflow obstruction** (pulmonary artery stenosis); **RVH**; and **"overriding" large ascending aorta**. Hypoxic spells with cyanosis may be life-threatening (brain damage). Tetralogy of Fallot is recognizable by cyanosis at or shortly after birth, by the characteristic x-ray findings, and by the pathognomonic **squatting episode** and **cyanotic spell**.

Epidemiology Tetralogy of Fallot is the **most common congenital cyanotic heart disease**. If left untreated, the mortality rate is 30% at 6 months and 90% to 95% at 20 years. After surgery, 85% of patients live 16 to 28 years.

Management Treat cyanotic spells with knee-chest position, oxygen, morphine, and beta-blockers. Evaluate with cardiac catheterization before surgical repair. Surgical repair consists of prosthetic closure of the VSD with restoration of RV outflow; **palliative surgery** consists of a shunt construction between the pulmonary and systemic (usually subclavian artery or thoracic aorta) arterial circulation. Pulmonary hypertension is the single most important determinant of success in surgery.

Complications CHF, ventricular arrhythmias, and sudden death.

Atlas Link UCVI PG-A-007

ID/CC	A 50-year-old **red-haired** man complains of **bleeding from a mole** located on his right arm.
HPI	Two months ago, he noticed that the lesion had **changed color and increased in size**. The patient works as a farmer (outdoor activity with **excessive sun exposure**).
PE	VS: normal. PE: **black-blue**, reticulated, **unevenly flecked**, hyper-pigmented lesion on posterolateral aspect of right arm; lesion has **irregular border** and small **satellite lesions** with a **raised, hyperkeratotic surface** and faint erythema around border; numerous actinic keratoses (a premalignant condition from sun exposure that may transform into squamous cell carcinoma) on forehead and back of hands; **axillary lymphadenopathy** noted.
Labs	CBC/Lytes/LFTs: normal. Punch **biopsy** reveals nodular melanoma.
Imaging	CXR: normal. Nuc: bone scan shows **metastases** to the humerus and pelvis. US/CT, liver: nodular solid masses compatible with metastatic disease.
Pathogenesis	Malignant melanoma is associated with exposure to **sunlight** (UV radiation), **genetic predisposition** (multiple lesions in families), and trauma (walking barefoot). The **ABCDEs** of melanoma are **asymmetry, border irregularity, color changes, diameter > 6 cm**, and **elevation**. Warning signs include the recent appearance of a nevus or a change in a preexisting skin lesion, itching, pain, ulceration, crusting, bleeding, and rapid growth. The chief complaint in blacks may be zones of vitiligo (initially). Common sites include the **back**, lower leg (in women), oral cavity, eye, anus, subungual area, soles of feet, CNS, and genitalia. There are four types. **Superficial spreading (most common), lentigo-maligna** (more common among the elderly), and **acral lentiginous** (affecting the palms, soles, and nail beds) all spread superficially and have a good prognosis. **Nodular melanoma**, however, exhibits rapid vertical growth (deeply invasive) and has a poor prognosis. **Prognosis and staging are based on tumor thickness (Breslow's), depth of invasion** (**Clark** level), **and location**. A poor prognosis is associated with lesions on the upper back, neck, posterolateral arm, and posterior scalp. Partial or complete regression may be seen.
Epidemiology	Melanoma constitutes **5% of skin cancers** and accounts for **two-thirds of all skin cancer deaths**. It is more common in **whites**,

MALIGNANT MELANOMA

with both sexes affected equally. Melanoma is increasing in incidence, with a mean age of 50. Two-thirds arise de novo; one-third arise from existing nevi (particularly the superficial spreading type). **Predisposing factors** include **congenital** and **dysplastic nevi** (premalignant; markers for increased risk of melanoma), blue eyes, **pale skin** (red-haired, albino), and pregnancy. The overall 5-year survival rate is 80%; with positive lymph nodes it is 30%, and with distant metastases 10%.

Management Workup includes **hepatic/bone scan**. Diagnose with punch or excisional **biopsy**. Treatment involves **surgery** with wide-margin excision, **chemotherapy** (dacarbazine, vinca alkaloids and cisplatin), and **immunotherapy** (interferon, interleukin, tumor-infiltrating lymphocyte). With < 0.75 mm invasion, prophylactic lymphadenectomy is not necessary. En bloc resection of superficial lymph nodes is performed for lymph node involvement. Sentinel node biopsies are useful in assessing lymphatic involvement.

Complications Metastatic disease (e.g., to the brain); poor prognosis in disseminated disease.

Atlas Link ⓊⒸⓋ2 SUR-004

MINICASE 335: BASAL CELL CARCINOMA

The most common skin cancer
- usually occurs in light-skinned people on sun-exposed areas
- presents with shiny, crusted ulcerations (RODENT ULCER), often with classic "pearly" rolled border and telangiectasias, slowly progressing in size
- treat by excision
- lesions rarely metastasize

Atlas Links: ⓊⒸⓋ2 MC-335A, MC-335B

MINICASE 336: EPIDERMAL INCLUSION CYST

Inflammation of a cyst
- presents with a tender, red, and rapidly enlarging nodule with white, cheesy exudates
- treat with incision and drainage

ID/CC A 24-year-old **obese** woman complains of a small **pulsating painful lump in her groin**.

HPI She first noticed the lump 6 days ago, developed a **fever 4** days ago, and today noticed a **yellowish discharge**. She works next to the oven in a pizza restaurant (continuous exposure to heat). She has undergone **periumbilical abscess drainage** and suffers from **acne**.

PE VS: **fever** (38.6°C). PE: no rashes; **cystic acne** on face, upper torso, and neck; no cervical lymphadenopathy; rounded, smooth, **hard, painful mass** in left groin with swollen, shiny surrounding skin, multiple fistulous tracts, and **pinpoint orifices** that exude **purulent greenish material**.

Labs CBC: **leukocytosis** (13,450/mm^3) **with 75% neutrophils**. Gram stain reveals **gram-positive cocci in "clusters of grapes"** (*Staphylococcus*); culture confirms staph.

Imaging XR, pelvis: normal; no evidence of bony involvement.

Pathogenesis Suppurative hidradenitis is a **chronic, indolent infection of the apocrine sweat glands**. With occlusion of glandular ducts, dilatation, subcutaneous infection, and abscess formation occur. It is most commonly caused by *Staphylococcus aureus*. *Streptococcus* and *Escherichia coli* species may be involved. The **initial stage involves pain, fever**, and **induration** (COLD ABSCESS), followed by **liquid pus with fluctuation** (MATURE ABSCESS) and spontaneous opening. The **late stage** is characterized by **multiple painful coalescent nodular abscesses** with surrounding skin **induration**.

Epidemiology Patients with **acne** or who are **obese**, continuously sweat, or are exposed to heat may develop hydradenitis. Most commonly located in the **axillae** (in females), **perineal region** (in males), areola of the nipple, and inframammary, inguinal, and periumbilical regions (areas of apocrine glands).

Management Prophylaxis consists of avoiding excessive sweating (induced by coffee, tea, and spicy foods) and local irritants (deodorants, talcum powder, shaving creams). In the cold abscess stage, **antibiotics** effective against *Staphylococcus* (e.g., cloxacillin) along with **hot compresses** are recommended. In the abscess stage, treatment consists of **surgical incision and drainage** at the point of maximal tension. Dressings should be changed frequently until

SUPPURATIVE HIDRADENITIS

there is no purulent drainage, at which time the wound may close secondarily. Recurrent, scarring disease may become chronic and indolent, warranting wide **excision of apocrine tissue** with skin grafting.

Complications   Suppurative phlebitis.

MINICASE 337: PORT-WINE STAIN

A mucosal skin lesion due to abnormal proliferation of superficial capillaries
- presents with large, sharply demarcated, purplish discoloration of the skin or mucous membranes of the face, mouth, or vagina
- if the lesion involves the vascular supply of the trigeminal nerve, seizures, hemiparesis, glaucoma, and mental retardation (STURGE–WEBER SYNDROME) result

---

ID/CC A 47-year-old **woman** presents with **chronic refractory hypertension**.

HPI She also complains of increased urinary frequency (POLYURIA), especially at night (NOCTURIA), and increased thirst (POLYDIPSIA). She additionally reports **profound muscle weakness and cramps** (due to hypokalemia), leg numbness and tingling (PARESTHESIAS), and recurrent **headaches**. She is not taking any potassium-wasting diuretics.

PE VS: normal HR; mild **diastolic hypertension** (BP 130/100). PE: minor diffuse retinal arteriolar narrowing (grade I hypertensive changes); no lymphadenopathy or JVD; regular rate and rhythm; no murmurs or rubs; abdominal exam normal with no bruits; slow DTRs; no pedal edema.

Labs Lytes: **hypernatremia**; hypomagnesemia; **hypokalemia**. ABGs: **metabolic alkalosis. Elevated plasma aldosterone; decreased renin** levels; elevated 24-hour urinary aldosterone and potassium; 2 L of normal saline infusion in 4 hours failed to suppress plasma aldosterone < 10 ng/dL; **glucose tolerance test abnormal**; renin-aldosterone stimulation (posture) test demonstrates decrease in aldosterone at 4 hours (vs. primary adrenocortical hyperplasia, in which there is an increase in aldosterone levels); load test with sodium produces hypokalemia. ECG: LVH (due to hypertension); flattening of T waves; prolonged QT interval, prominent U waves (secondary to hypokalemia).

Imaging **[A]** MR: small left **adrenal mass (1)**; adrenal vein catheterization shows **ipsilateral (left-sided) elevation of aldosterone**; note the kidney (K) and pancreas (P).

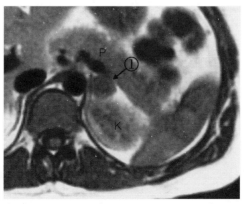

[A]

HYPERALDOSTERONISM—PRIMARY

Pathogenesis	The **most common cause** of hyperaldosteronism is **Conn's syndrome**, an adrenocortical adenoma that is usually single and unilateral and that produces increased aldosterone, a potent mineralocorticoid. Other causes include **primary adrenocortical hyperplasia** and **adrenal cancer** (rare). Hyperaldosteronism typically involves the **triad of hypertension, hypokalemia, and low renin**. Unlike essential hypertension, hypertension secondary to Conn's syndrome is unresponsive to ACE inhibitors. Elevated serum aldosterone causes hypokalemia, increased urinary excretion of potassium, and hypernatremia (mediated by its effect on the distal renal tubule).
Epidemiology	Primary hyperaldosteronism causes less than 1% of cases of hypertension and is more common in **females**.
Management	The aldosterone antagonist **spironolactone** is used to control hypertension and hypokalemia. Treatment of an aldosterone-producing adenoma consists of **unilateral adrenalectomy**. Hypoaldosteronism (hyperkalemia, hypotension) may ensue several days postoperatively (due to long-standing suppression of the contralateral adrenal). **In bilateral adrenal hyperplasia**, treatment consists of spironolactone, antihypertensive drugs, and dexamethasone suppression.
Complications	Renal damage, MI, and stroke secondary to chronic hypertension; rhabdomyolysis, arrhythmias, and paralysis from hypokalemia; and carpopedal spasm/tetany due to alkalosis.

MINICASE 338: HYPERTHYROIDISM (SOLITARY NODULE)

The most common thyroid neoplasm, much more common in females than in males
- presents with a solitary thyroid nodule
- nuclear scan reveals cold nodule
- treat with surgical excision

Atlas Link: U C V 1 PG-P1-054

ID/CC A 32-year-old man complains of **facial flushing** that began following a stressful business meeting; he also complains of recurring severe, throbbing **headaches** (due to increased BP).

he has been suffering from **episodic nausea,** ıitations, and **anxiety**. He also acknowledges ı and a **weight loss** of 5 kg over the past ırrently asymptomatic. He denies drug use cations.

C); **hypertension** (BP 210/125); normal HR. ımias; abdominal exam normal.

ıes (epinephrine/norepinephrine) elevated ıst; **clonidine** fails to significantly suppress ıes; **elevated glucose** (due to increased cate- ʌated 24-hour **vanillylmandelic acid** (VMA). ɔcolate, and medications may artificially

e **right adrenal mass. [B]** MR, abdomen: lateral adrenal masses. **[C]** Nuc, MIBG: ased left adrenal activity.

idiopathic primary neoplasms of the drenal medulla (derived from **embryonic** ːing **epinephrine and norepinephrine**. the retroperitoneal, pelvic, or cervical ;ympathetic nervous system. While ʌsent a treatable cause of **persistent** ney may also produce **transient,** ..are instances, ACTH may be secreted аг∪ produce bilateral adrenal hyperplasia and Cushing's syndrome.

Epidemiology Constitutes 0.2% of patients with hypertension and is the **most common adrenal medullary tumor in adults. The rule of 10s** applies: 10% malignant, 10% bilateral, 10% extra-adrenal, 10% calcify, 10% familial, and 10% children. Pheochromocytomas may be a part of **MEN IIa (Sipple's) syndrome** (pheochromocytoma, medullary carcinoma of the thyroid, and parathyroid adenoma) and **MEN IIb syndrome** (pheochromocytoma, medullary thyroid carcinoma, and oral and intestinal ganglioneuromatosis) as well as von Hippel–Lindau disease and neurofibromatosis. Isolated pheochromocytomas may also occur in a familial pattern.

7 **PHEOCHROMOCYTOMA**

Epicurean and Company
3800 Reservoir Rd. NW
202-625-2222

Party of 1
Customer Receipt   Ticket   4002
able   4002   REG1
erver   : Krista   Date 08/07/09
1:15 AM

1.00 Pizza   3.25
      Pz] Single Slice

              Sub Total   :   3.25
              Sales Tax   :   .33
           Check Total $ 3.58
                             3.58
           Cash
           Change Due   :   .00

Thank you. Please come again.

Management **Blood pressure control** with **phenoxybenzamine or prazosin** (alpha blockade) for 1 to 3 weeks prior to surgery. Chronic volume contraction is controlled with liberal salt intake. **Beta-blockers** are useful in preventing catecholamine-induced arrhythmias and tachycardia, but only after adequate peripheral vasodilation with alpha blockade. **Surgical resection** follows α-adrenergic blockade. Close intra- and postoperative hemodynamic **monitoring** is indicated to prevent the profound postresection hypotension that results from peripheral vasodilation.

Complications Cardiac and cerebral damage due to malignant hypertension, cardiomyopathy, CHF, and metastatic disease.

Atlas Links 󰚛󰚛󰚛󰚛 PG-BC-026A, PG-BC-026B, PM-BC-026

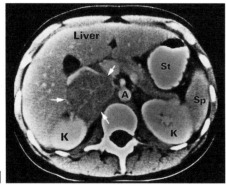
[A]

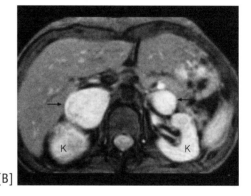
[B]

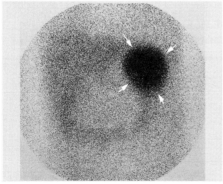
[C]

ID/CC	A 24-year-old woman complains of a **painless mass in the anterior portion of her neck**.
HPI	The mass has been present for 2 years but did not exhibit growth until recently. As a child in South America, she received **radiotherapy** to the neck for tuberculous adenitis. She denies any dysphonia, dysphagia, or dyspnea.
PE	VS: normal. PE: well developed and nourished; **solitary**, non-tender, rounded **hard mass on right lobe of thyroid** gland that displaces as gland moves with swallowing; discrete **cervical adenopathy**; normal breast, lung, and skin exams.
Labs	Calcium, alkaline phosphatase, and serum calcitonin normal (increased in medullary carcinoma of the thyroid); **TFTs normal**. FNA and cytology show **papillary thyroid cancer with psammoma bodies**.
Imaging	CXR: normal (to rule out substernal extension or lung metastases). US: **solid right lobe thyroid mass**. **[A]** Nuc (Tc-99 pertechnetate isotope): **hypofunctional** (COLD) nodule in the right lobe.

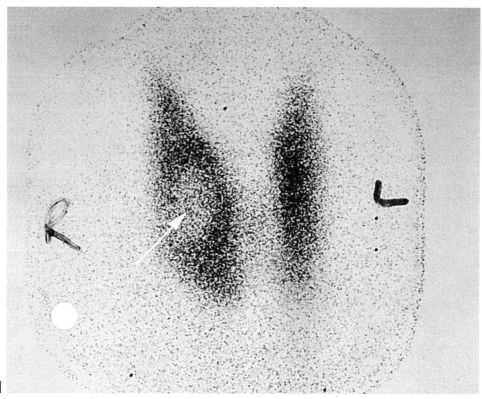

[A]

THYROID CARCINOMA

Pathogenesis Thyroid neoplasms are **carcinomas (papillary, follicular, sclerosing, medullary, or anaplastic)** or **lymphomas**. Patients are usually asymptomatic and **euthyroid**; the presenting complaint is often a **painless thyroid nodule** or **adenopathy**. Malignancy is suggested by a **solitary nodule** (vs. multinodular goiter), fixation, rapid growth, vocal cord paralysis, hoarseness, hard consistency, and fixed adenopathy. **Cold nodules** (vs. functional or warm ones) are **more likely to be malignant**. Previous **neck irradiation** for skin and lymph node pathology greatly increases the risk of papillary thyroid cancer. Male gender, young and old age, and a history of thyroiditis are other risk factors.

Epidemiology Four percent of the U.S. adult population have palpable nodules, fewer than 5% of which are malignant. **Papillary** is the most common type, is seen in young adults, and is characterized by early lymphatic metastasis and **slow growth** (most benign variety). It has an 80% 10-year survival rate. The **follicular** type affects an older age group, has a more rubbery consistency, and disseminates hematogenously to bones and lungs; metastases take up radioactive iodine. The **mixed** (papillary-follicular) type behaves like papillary cancer. The **medullary** type arises in the parafollicular C cells, runs in families, is associated with MEN IIa and IIb syndromes, and produces calcitonin. **Undifferentiated forms** (ANAPLASTIC; small, giant, and spindle-cell forms) affect older women, are rapidly infiltrating, and carry a poor prognosis. Prognosis depends not only on type but on extension and DNA ploidy.

Management Treatment for **papillary** carcinoma is **total thyroidectomy**. If there is gross lymph node involvement, a conservative modified radical neck dissection should be performed. For **follicular** or **medullary** carcinoma, **total thyroidectomy** is necessary (due to multicentricity); if lymph nodes are positive, a modified radical neck dissection must be performed. Metastases are treated with **radioactive iodine. Thyroglobulin** is a useful tumor marker because it rises if there is residual or recurrent tumor. **Undifferentiated** carcinomas call for **thyroidectomy, radiotherapy**, and **chemotherapy** (doxorubicin, vincristine, chlorambucil).

Complications Metastatic disease, vocal cord paralysis, and hypocalcemia (can be seen in medullary thyroid carcinoma secondary to calcitonin secretion by tumor cells).

Atlas Link ⬚U⬚C⬚V⬚I⬚ PM-P1-061

ID/CC	A 40-year-old **morbidly obese** man presents with severe **daytime sleepiness** (SOMNOLENCE) and morning headaches.
HPI	Directed questioning reveals **hypnagogic hallucinations** (vividly colored dreams mixed with sensory perceptions) and nightmares; his libido has also decreased. His wife reports that he **snores heavily** with periods of silence (apnea) during the night. The patient also reports that although he naps 3 to 4 times per day, he never feels refreshed. He has also fallen asleep while driving on two occasions. He denies cataplexy or sleep paralysis associated with narcolepsy.
PE	VS: **hypertension** (BP 150/90). PE: morbidly **obese** (380 lb); voice has nasal twang; **retrognathia; oropharynx narrowed** by excessive soft tissue; large tonsils; pendulous uvula and prominent tongue (MACROGLOSSIA); cardiac auscultation reveals **loud P$_2$** (from pulmonary hypertension).
Labs	CBC: hematocrit 50%. TFTs normal. ECG: RVH. Polysomnography reveals **> 5 apneic spells** lasting 1 to 2 minutes each hour with O$_2$ saturation dropping to as low as 80% during episodes.
Imaging	CXR: large pulmonary arteries and redistribution of pulmonary blood flow. Echo: RVH and dilatation.
Pathogenesis	Relaxation of the upper airway during sleep can cause respiratory airway collapse and obstruction with resulting apnea in patients with structural narrowing of the upper airway. The consequences of chronic hypoxemia include pulmonary hypertension, cor pulmonale, CHF, secondary erythrocytosis, and cardiac arrhythmias.
Epidemiology	Most commonly affects **middle-age, obese males**. Other causes of **anatomic narrowing** of the upper airways (e.g., tonsillar hypertrophy, obesity, macroglossia, micrognathia) also predispose.
Management	**Weight reduction** has been shown to improve breathing. Avoiding alcohol and sedative medications at night is also helpful. The most effective and frequently applied therapy is nasal **continuous positive airway pressure (CPAP)** at night. Refractory cases may demand surgical treatment with **uvulopalatopharyngoplasty**.
Complications	Complications include systemic hypertension, LVH, ischemic heart disease, pulmonary hypertension, cor pulmonale, and respiratory failure. Unexpected death during sleep may result from MI, arrhythmias, and asphyxia.

OBSTRUCTIVE SLEEP APNEA

ID/CC A **48-year-old** man complains of **difficulty swallowing both solid and liquid foods** (DYSPHAGIA) and a 7-kg **weight loss** over 9 months.

HPI He states that he frequently **regurgitates** undigested food, especially at night. His dysphagia has **slowly progressed** in severity and frequency over the past year.

PE VS: normal. PE: **thin; bad breath** (HALITOSIS); abdominal exam unremarkable.

Labs **Low albumin** (poor nutrition); **ANA** negative; **endoscopy** (to exclude carcinoma) reveals stagnation of food and marked dilatation of esophagus; no strictures; lower esophageal sphincter (LES) hypertonic; biopsy rules out carcinoma; **manometry** reveals **high intraesophageal resting pressure, increased LES pressure**, loss of normal peristaltic waves, and **inadequate LES relaxation after swallow.**

Imaging **[A]** and **[B]** UGI: **marked esophageal dilatation** (1) (MEGAESOPHAGUS); **absent LES relaxation** and disorganized peristaltic

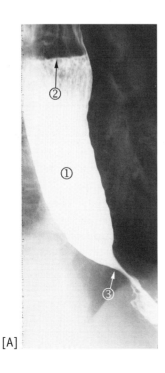
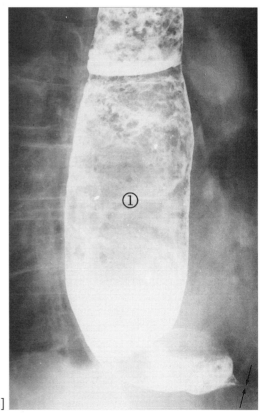

[A]   [B]

contractions; **air-fluid level** (2) in the proximal esophagus; **"bird's-beak" or "rat-tail" narrowing** (3) of the distal esophagus.

Pathogenesis Achalasia results from **impaired inhibitory innervation of Auerbach's plexus,** causing defective LES relaxation. Pathogenic theories include a lesion of the dorsal vagus motor nucleus by a neurotropic virus or an esophageal hypersensitivity to gastrin. Achalasia may also present as a paraneoplastic process in older individuals. Also called **cardiospasm,** it characteristically presents with **high LES resting pressure** and **absence of peristaltic contractions** in the body of the esophagus, causing **dysphagia, particularly to cold liquids**.

Epidemiology Achalasia is an uncommon disease (6 in 100,000) that usually occurs in middle age.

Management Medical management of mild cases with oral nitrates or calcium channel blockers. Many cases resolve with **balloon dilatation** (beware of perforation). Endoscopic **botulinum toxin injection** into the LES may relieve the obstruction for up to a year. In long-standing disease with marked tortuosity, a Heller **cardiomyotomy** (esophageal muscle incision at the cardioesophageal junction) is effective but can result in gastroesophageal regurgitation; treat with proton pump inhibitors. Long-term follow-up is necessary after any treatment modality (cancer may develop years later).

Complications Complications include esophageal carcinoma, aspiration pneumonia, abscess, bronchiectasis, pulmonary fibrosis, esophageal ulcerations, and malnutrition. Postsurgical esophageal reflux may result in esophagitis and hemorrhage if untreated.

MINICASE 339: BOERHAAVE'S SYNDROME

Postemetic rupture of the esophagus
- common in bulimia and pregnancy
- presents with retrosternal pain after vigorous vomiting, tachycardia, possible hypoaerated lung, and mediastinal emphysema
- UGI shows extravasation of contrast into the mediastinum, esophagoscopy shows complete rupture of the wall
- treat with broad-spectrum antibiotics (to prevent mediastinal infection) and surgical repair

ID/CC	A 68-year-old man complains of dull, achy **left lower quadrant abdominal pain** with fever, chills, and malaise of 3 days' duration.
HPI	He also complains of recent alternating diarrhea and constipation and increased urinary frequency. He is a chain smoker and consumes a **low-fiber, high-fat diet**.
PE	VS: **tachycardia** (HR 110); normal BP; **fever** (38.3°C). PE: mild dehydration; mild abdominal distention with **left lower quadrant tenderness**; localized voluntary muscle **guarding**; discrete oblong **mass** in left lower quadrant; bowel sounds diminished; rectal exam reveals hemorrhoids; heme-positive stool.
Labs	CBC: decreased hemoglobin (10 gm/dL); leukocytosis (16,300/mm^3) with neutrophilia (78%) and **18% bands** (left shift). UA/Lytes: normal.
Imaging	CXR: **free intraperitoneal subdiaphragmatic air** (perforation of hollow viscus [sigmoid colon] walled off). KUB: small bowel loop dilatation; increased radiodensity in the left lower quadrant. CT: blurring of pericolic fat; **mass in the wall of the sigmoid colon**. **[A]** BE: many barium-filled diverticula are seen throughout the colon in another patient (**barium enemas are contraindicated in acute diverticulitis** because of the risk of leakage and severe peritonitis). **[B]** BE: an abscess is seen in another patient resulting from diverticular disease. **[C]** BE: barium can be seen entering the bladder (1) in this patient with a colovesicular fistula (2).
Pathogenesis	Diverticula are **herniations** of the mucosa and submucosa through the muscular layers of the bowel wall (FALSE DIVERTICULUM) and result from **high intraluminal pressures**. These herniations usually arise at **sites where arterioles traverse the colonic wall** and thus are prone to bleed. These outpouchings may also be obstructed, permitting unabated growth of bacteria and consequent inflammation (DIVERTICULITIS). Diverticulitis has a higher incidence in the left colon (rectosigmoid region) than elsewhere in the GI tract and is **most common in the sigmoid**, where intraluminal pressures are highest. Diverticulitis classically presents as **"left-sided appendicitis."**
Epidemiology	Colonic diverticula occur predominantly in **those older than 70 years**. Risk factors include a **low-fiber diet**, as seen in

11   DIVERTICULITIS

developed countries. Perforation and consequent generalized peritonitis occur in 10% to 15% of patients.

Management Treat with **IV fluids, NPO**, and **antibiotics** effective against gram-positive, gram-negative, and anaerobic organisms (e.g., ciprofloxacin plus metronidazole). After an acute episode, a colonic evaluation is needed (one-third of patients have a colonic tumor). Long-term management involves **increased dietary fiber intake** and regular exercise. In cases of recurrent diverticulitis (10% after a single uncomplicated episode and > 30% otherwise), patients should consider sigmoidectomy. **Surgery** is indicated in the presence of an abscess (that cannot be drained percutaneously), generalized peritonitis, a fistula, an obstruction, or failure of medical therapy.

Complications Infection may cause necrosis of the colonic wall with **perforation** (microscopically or macroscopically), abscess formation, or peritonitis. Other complications include **obstruction** and **fistula**.

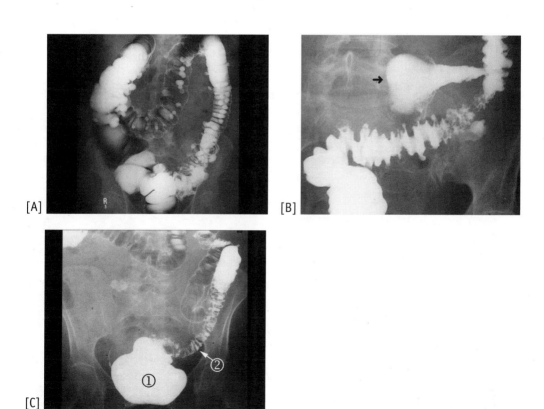

[A]   [B]   [C]

ID/CC A **42-year-old man** complains of dull, persistent epigastric pain.

HPI For 2 days he has had fever without chills along with nausea and scant vomiting. Two weeks ago, he was hospitalized for acute gallstone pancreatitis.

PE VS: **fever** (38.5°C); hypertension (BP 140/80); tachycardia (HR 110). PE: alert, active, and in no acute distress; moderate tenderness and a palpable, deep-seated, immotile **mass in epigastric area**; no peritoneal signs.

Labs CBC: moderate **leukocytosis** (15,200/mm³) **with neutrophilia. Mildly elevated blood glucose; hyperamylasemia**; elevated serum lipase.

Imaging US: **fluid-filled mass** adjacent to the pancreas. **[A]** CT, abdomen: fluid-filled cyst (1) originating in the pancreatic tail. **[B]** CT, abdomen: a different case with a large unilocular pseudocyst (1). **[C]** CT, abdomen: another case with a hemorrhagic perisplenic pseudocyst. **[D]** CT, abdomen: a different case with both a large lesser sac pseudocyst (1) and a small intrapancreatic pseudocyst (2).

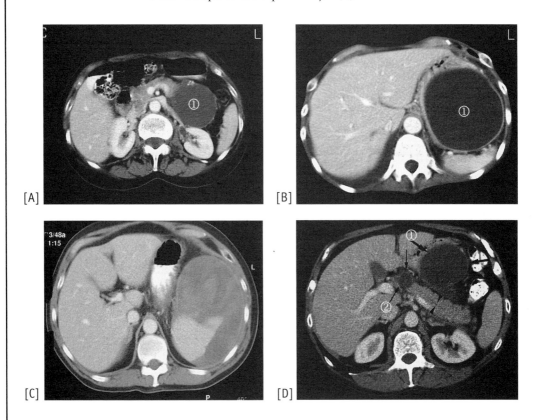

[A] [B] [C] [D]

Pathogenesis	Most pancreatic pseudocysts occur **following attacks of acute pancreatitis**, when pancreatic juices fill areas of glandular necrosis, forming compartments of sterile fluid that persist even as inflammation diminishes. Infection of these compartments causes pancreatic abscesses. Pseudocysts **lack an epithelial lining** while frequently containing high concentrations of pancreatic enzymes. Pseudocysts may also be caused by trauma (most common cause of pseudocysts in children), surgical procedures, and alcohol damage. Pseudocysts are **usually single**.
Epidemiology	Three percent of patients with acute pancreatitis develop a pseudocyst.
Management	Cysts > 5 cm should be drained after being allowed to **mature 6 weeks. Internal drainage** (anastomosis to internal viscus) is performed most commonly. **Percutaneous drainage** is preferred for infected cysts. Small cysts (< 5 cm) **often regress spontaneously**.
Complications	**Rupture** produces peritonitis and is associated with a high mortality. Pseudocysts usually grow rapidly before rupturing. **Infection and bleeding** (intracystic—enlarging mass; intragastric—hematemesis; intraperitoneal—shock) may also occur.

MINICASE 340: COLONIC POLYPS

Projection of intestinal mucosa into the lumen of the colon
- causes vary and include inflammatory, hyperplastic, and neoplastic processes
- present with asymptomatic occult bleeding (although larger lesions may cause alteration in bowel habits), increased stool frequency, change in stool caliber, constipation, and tenesmus
- stool hemoccult cards are intermittently positive for occult blood
- colonoscopy shows polyps, with pathology determining the etiology
- treat with polypectomy, surgical resection with adjunctive chemotherapy depending on the polyps' pathology

ID/CC	A 56-year-old man is admitted for severe **midepigastric** abdominal pain that **radiates to the back**.
HPI	The **pain improves** when the patient **assumes the fetal position** or **leans forward** and worsens with deep breathing and movement. He also complains of **anorexia, nausea, vomiting**, and **syncope**. The patient is an **alcoholic** and spent the past 3 days binge drinking.
PE	VS: **tachycardia** (HR 110); tachypnea (RR 28); **fever** (38.6°C); **hypotension** (BP 90/60). PE: agitated and **confused**; dry mucous membranes; decreased breath sounds over left lower lung; **abdomen tender and distended with diminished bowel sounds**; voluntary **guarding** in upper abdomen; mild rigidity without rebound tenderness; ecchymotic discoloration of periumbilical skin (CULLEN'S SIGN) and over both flanks (GREY–TURNER'S SIGN); facial muscle spasm when facial nerve is tapped (CHVOSTEK'S SIGN for hypocalcemia); carpopedal spasm when blood pressure cuff is applied (TROUSSEAU'S SIGN for hypocalcemia).
Labs	**Markedly increased serum and urinary amylase and lipase**. Five of the following **Ranson's criteria** present: (1) **on admission**: age > 55, leukocytosis > 16,000/mm³, glucose > 200, LDH > 350, AST > 250. (2) **At 48 hours**: > 10% hematocrit decrease; > 5 mg% increase in BUN, calcium < 8, hypoxemia < 60, base deficit > 4, fluid sequestration > 6 L (3 to 4 signs = 20% mortality; 5 to 6 signs = 40% mortality; > 7 signs = 100% mortality).
Imaging	CXR: small left **pleural effusion**; basal **atelectasis**. KUB: localized ileus (SENTINEL LOOP); gas in the ascending but not in the transverse colon (COLON CUTOFF SIGN). **[A]** CT, abdomen (diagnostic procedure of choice): edema of the pancreas; peripancreatic stranding. **[B]** A different case with peripancreatic fluid collection. **[C]** CT, abdomen: for comparison, a case of chronic pancreatitis with pancreatic atrophy and calcification.
Pathogenesis	Pancreatitis is caused mainly by **alcohol abuse** and **gallstones**. Other causes include hyperlipidemia, hypercalcemia, pancreatic tumors, parasitic obstructions (ascaris), collagen vascular diseases, CMV infection (in HIV-positive patients), Legionnaire's disease, *Campylobacter*, viral infections, steroids, other medications, and trauma (ERCP, stomach and gallbladder surgery). Approximately 10% of cases are idiopathic. In gallstone pancreatitis, bile reflux, spasm, or obstruction of the ampulla of Vater may lead to enzyme activation inside the gland with **autodigestion**. Physical signs do not always reflect the severity of the disease.

13 **PANCREATITIS—ACUTE**

Epidemiology Annually, between three and six individuals in 10,000 are affected, and the incidence appears to be increasing. Alcohol and biliary disease account for 90% of patients.

Management Patients should be **NPO** with **nasogastric suction**. Maintain fluid and electrolyte balance; control pain with **meperidine**. Give **total parenteral nutrition** if NPO > 7 days. Give **antibiotics** if infected bile is suspected. With signs of necrosis, peripancreatic drainage, continuous pancreatic irrigation, subtotal pancreatectomy, or peritoneal lavage may be indicated. In gallstone pancreatitis, a cholecystectomy is indicated after the pancreatitis resolves. **Pseudocyst**: if < 6 weeks, observe (40% resolve alone); if > 6 weeks, open internal drainage. **Abscess**: drain externally via tubes or open-wound technique with lavage under anesthesia every 2 days (Bradley's).

Complications DIC, renal failure, systemic sepsis, multiorgan systemic failure, toxic psychosis, lactic acidosis, pseudocyst, abscess, septicemia, subcutaneous fat necrosis, and pancreatic exocrine and endocrine insufficiency.

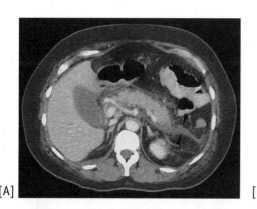

[A]

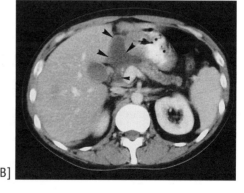

[B]

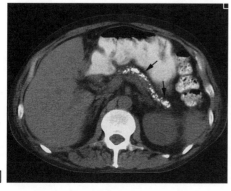

[C]

MINICASE 341: HIATAL HERNIA

Intrathoracic protrusion of part of the stomach through the diaphragmatic hiatus
- the sliding type commonly causes reflux, whereas the paraesophageal type causes pressure symptoms
- presents with retrosternal pain that worsens when the patient assumes a supine position as well as with regurgitation of sour material
- more common with smoking, alcohol, and obesity
- UGI shows the gastroesophageal junction and part of the stomach protruding above the diaphragm
- treat with weight loss, cessation of tobacco and alcohol use, avoidance of the supine position following meals, prokinetics, H_2 blockers, proton pump inhibitors, surgery
- complications include Barrett's esophagus, erosive and ulcerative esophagitis, peptic stricture, GI hemorrhage, incarceration and obstruction

MINICASE 342: TOXIC MEGACOLON

Extreme dilatation of the large bowel that can be congenital in Hirschsprung's disease or acquired due to ulcerative colitis, pseudomembranous colitis, or Chagas' disease
- presents with fever, severe abdominal pain, rebound tenderness, and rigid abdomen
- AXR reveals marked colonic dilatation with obstructive signs (e.g., air-fluid levels, lack of air in the rectum)
- treat according to cause (e.g., metronidazole for pseudomembranous colitis), surgical resection of bowel
- complications include perforation, sepsis, and death

ID/CC A 37-year-old **male** CEO presents with **severe epigastric pain** and **nausea**.

HPI He **vomited** today and has a 2-week history of intermittent epigastric pain radiating to the back that is relieved by food. He works under a great deal of **stress** and drinks six cups of **coffee** and one fifth of **alcohol** each day. He also **smokes** two packs of cigarettes a day (30-pack-year history) and takes **aspirin** on a regular basis.

PE VS: **fever** (38.7°C); tachycardia (HR 115); **hypotension** (BP 90/50); tachypnea. PE: in **acute distress; diaphoretic**; mild pallor; **abdomen rigid with generalized tenderness** and positive **rebound**; bowel sounds absent; heme-positive stools on rectal exam.

Labs CBC: hemoglobin 12.1 gm/dL; **leukocytosis** (18,400/mm³) **with 85% neutrophils**. Amylase mildly elevated; *Helicobacter pylori* serum antibodies present.

Imaging **[A]** CXR: **free subdiaphragmatic intraperitoneal air (1) (perforated viscus)**. **[B]** UGI: a different case showing a giant gastric ulcer (1) with radiating mucosal folds. **[C]** UGI: another case showing an outpouching from the lesser curvature.

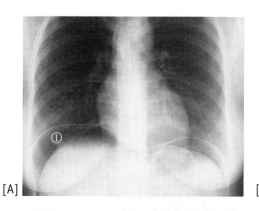

[A]

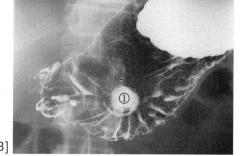

[B]

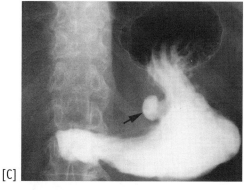

[C]

PEPTIC ULCER—PERFORATED

Pathogenesis Ulcers occur when the mucosal barrier is eroded. They result from decreased mucosal resistance, as occurs in **H. pylori** infection and **aspirin and NSAID** use. Ulcers are associated with smoking, alcohol, and steroid use. Duodenal ulcers are associated with acid hypersecretion, whereas gastric ulcers are not. Lesions are **usually single** and in 85% of cases are in the **duodenum** (usually within 2 cm of the pylorus); 15% of cases occur in the stomach (usually in the lesser curvature). Lesions may also be found in a gastrojejunal stoma and Meckel's diverticulum. Duodenal ulcers generally affect younger patients, whereas gastric ulcers occur in older patients, with pain occurring earlier after meals. A complication may be the first manifestation; alternatively, only vague dyspeptic symptoms may be seen.

Epidemiology More frequently affects **males**, those with blood group O, patients with chronic liver and lung disease, and individuals with diets high in carbohydrates and protein but low in fiber. The incidence of the disease and its complications is decreasing (due to proton pump inhibitors and antibiotics for *H. pylori*).

Management Perforation of a gastric ulcer requires a partial gastrectomy and vagotomy, while perforation of a duodenal ulcer requires closure of the perforation, pyloroplasty, and vagotomy. If the patient is critical and the ulcer is gastric, treat via closure with an omental patch (GRAHAM'S PATCH). **Bleeding** resolves in 75% of cases without operation. *H. pylori*-associated ulcer disease is treated with a combination of a 10- to 14-day, two- or three-antibiotic regimen combined with a proton pump inhibitor for 4 to 8 weeks. Prostaglandin analogs and sucralfate can be used to protect GI mucosa. Active uncomplicated ulcers are treated with proton pump inhibitors or H_2 receptor blockers alone.

Complications Complications include **gastric outlet obstruction**, hemorrhage, and malignant change associated with gastric ulcers. Postoperative complications include leakage, hemorrhage, postvagotomy diarrhea, fistula, stomal ulcer, alkaline gastritis, blind loop syndrome, dumping syndrome, and iron and vitamin B_{12} deficiency.

Atlas Links ☐☐☐☐☐ PG-A-024A, PG-A-024B

ID/CC   A **45-year-old white woman** presents with **difficulty swallowing** (DYSPHAGIA) for the past 2 weeks.

HPI   She states that she **tires easily** while performing daily activities and has experienced a 10-kg weight loss over the past 4 months. She is a **Norwegian** immigrant with a strange **craving for ice and clay** (PICA; due to iron deficiency).

PE   VS: mild **tachycardia**. PE: **pale; edentulous; atrophic oral mucosa**; tongue smooth and shiny red (GLOSSITIS); fissures at angle of mouth (CHEILOSIS); mild splenomegaly; **spoon-shaped fingernails** (KOILONYCHIA).

Labs   CBC: low hemoglobin and MCV; **microcytic anemia**; thrombocytopenia; normal reticulocyte count. **Low serum iron; decreased ferritin; increased TIBC.**

Imaging   [A] UGI: small web at C5 level.

Pathogenesis   Also called Patterson-Kelly syndrome, Plummer–Vinson syndrome consists of single or multiple concentric **esophageal webs** that

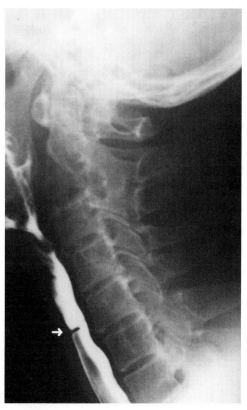

[A]

PLUMMER–VINSON SYNDROME

produce **dysphagia**. These webs are associated with **severe iron deficiency** and anemia and can be accompanied by other iron deficiency stigmata, such as cheilosis, atrophic glossitis, and spooning of the nails. Ten percent of Plummer-Vinson patients ultimately develop **squamous cell carcinoma of the esophagus**, hypopharynx, or oral cavity.

Epidemiology   The disease is generally seen in edentulous middle-aged **women**. It has an increased frequency in people of **Scandinavian and British origin**.

Management   **Esophageal dilatation** with mercury-filled tubes (BOUGIENAGE) coupled with **iron supplementation** is the mainstay of therapy. An upper GI series and endoscopy with biopsy should be done in all patients.

Complications   Increased incidence of **esophageal and pharyngeal cancer**.

ID/CC	A 41-year-old man was found on the floor in a **confused and stuporous** state (altered mental status) with "especially bad breath" (ammonia).
HPI	The patient is a **chronic alcoholic** who binges three to five times a week. His neighbor reports that he **vomited blood** (HEMATEMESIS; due to esophageal varices) 2 days ago. He has also complained of **severe hemorrhoids**.
PE	VS: no fever; tachycardia (HR 105); hypotension (BP 90/60); no orthopnea; mild tachypnea (RR 20). PE: obtunded, disheveled, and disoriented; dehydrated and mildly **jaundiced; no JVD; parotid enlargement**; fine **flapping tremor of hands** with extension (ASTERIXIS); **spider angiomata; gynecomastia**; muscle wasting; **palmar erythema; caput medusae**; nodular, hard liver palpable 4 cm below costal margin; **bulging, dull flanks** and fluid wave (ASCITES); **splenomegaly; testicular atrophy**; pitting pedal edema.
Labs	CBC: macrocytic, hypochromic **anemia** (Hb 7.1 gm/dL); **thrombocytopenia**. LFTs: **AST/ALT ratio 2:1** (alcoholic hepatic damage); **elevated PT, transaminases, GGT, and alkaline phosphatase. Blood glucose low; high blood ammonia**; increased aromatic and decreased branched chain amino acids; **hypoalbuminemia**; liver biopsy diagnostic of cirrhosis of liver (if contraindicated, do peritoneoscopy).
Imaging	**[A]** UGI: filling defects in **"string of beads"** pattern (esophageal varices). Endoscopy: confirms grade III varices and is therapeutic (sclerotherapy). **[B]** CT, abdomen: a different case with a heterogeneous liver and large recanalized umbilical vein.
Pathogenesis	The etiologies of elevated portal venous pressure (> 10 mmHg) are classified as prehepatic, intrahepatic, and posthepatic. **Intrahepatic** causes include **cirrhosis** (alcoholic, postnecrotic, biliary), hepatitis B and C, hemochromatosis, Wilson's disease, and schistosomiasis; **prehepatic** causes include portal venous occlusion via thrombosis or extrinsic compression; and **posthepatic** causes include constrictive pericarditis and hepatic vein obstruction (Budd-Chiari syndrome). **Collateral circulation develops in an effort to decompress the portal system**, and **portosystemic anastomoses** are formed as follows: left gastric → azygous (**esophageal varices**); superior → middle and inferior rectal veins (**hemorrhoids**); paraumbilical → inferior gastric (**caput medusae**). Of the many collaterals formed secondary to portal hypertension, bleeding is rare except from esophageal varices. Half of all such patients die from this acute event.

GASTROENTEROLOGY

Management   Establish **hemodynamic stability**. Treat variceal bleeding with **sclerotherapy** (may cause ulceration and stricture), **octreotide** or **vasopressin**, and **balloon tamponade** (Sengstaken–Blakemore tube). **Surgical shunts** between the portal and systemic circulation decrease portal hypertension but may precipitate encephalopathy. Other treatment modalities include **transjugular intrahepatic portosystemic shunt (TIPS)**, splenectomy, devascularization of the lower esophagus (SUGIURA), and **liver transplantation**. Treatment of hepatic encephalopathy includes searching for precipitating factors (dehydration, medications, GI bleed, constipation), reduction of dietary protein, and administration of **neomycin** and/or **lactulose** (to decrease ammonia absorption).

Complications   Massive hemorrhage (secondary to ruptured esophageal varices), ascites, spontaneous bacterial peritonitis, hepatic encephalopathy, portal vein thrombosis, hypersplenism, and hemorrhoids.

Atlas Link   ⬚Ｕ|Ｃ|Ｖ|１⬚ PG-A-025

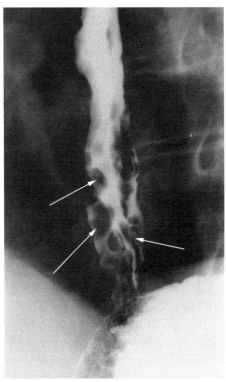

[A]

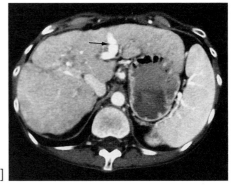

[B]

ID/CC	A **41-year-old black woman** presents with **right upper quadrant abdominal pain** associated with **nausea** and **vomiting** that began after she ate an egg-and-avocado salad (fatty foods).
HPI	She states that the pain **radiates to the right scapular region** (referred pain) and also acknowledges nausea and one episode of vomiting. This is the third time such pain has brought this **mother of four** (MULTIPAROUS) to the ER; previous episodes were less intense and spontaneously regressed within a few hours.
PE	VS: tachycardia; fever (38.6°C). PE: **obese**; marked tenderness in right upper quadrant with **localized guarding**; gallbladder palpable in subcostal region (30% of cases); **sudden inspiratory arrest** with palpation of right subcostal region (MURPHY'S SIGN).
Labs	CBC: **leukocytosis** (15,500/mm^3) **with neutrophilia** (83%). Elevated ESR. LFTs: bilirubin and alkaline phosphatase slightly elevated; AST and ALT normal; amylase normal.
Imaging	**[A]** US (diagnostic procedure of choice for cholelithiasis): **thickening of the gallbladder wall** (1) **with gallstones** (2). HIDA (gallbladder is imaged; diagnostic procedure of choice for acute cholecystitis): shows no uptake of radionuclide in gallbladder. **[B]** XR, abdomen: a different case showing multiple radiopaque gallstones (seen in only 15% of cases). **[C]** US: another case showing acalculous cholecystitis (wall thickening with no stones).
Pathogenesis	Acute cholecystitis generally results from **obstruction of the gallbladder neck or cystic duct by an impacted stone**, leading to ischemia, ulceration, edema, inflammation, and bacterial infection (common organisms include *Escherichia coli*, *Klebsiella*, and enterococcus). There are three types of stones: cholesterol (approximately 75%), black pigment (associated with hemolysis or cirrhosis), and brown pigment (associated with infection). The three steps in cholesterol gallstone formation are cholesterol saturation, nucleation, and growth. Typically, pain starts after a fatty meal (stimulation of gallbladder contraction leads to impaction of stone in cystic duct or Hartmann's pouch, which leads to blockage of bile exit). Murphy's sign, fever, and leukocytosis suggest a diagnosis of cholecystitis rather than simple biliary colic. **Acalculous** (NO STONES) **cholecystitis** is found in patients with severe debilitating diseases, burns, sepsis, and parasitic (ascariasis) or bacterial (typhoid fever) infections and, less commonly, in those on a prolonged fast or on total parenteral nutrition.

ACUTE CHOLECYSTITIS

Epidemiology The prototypical patient displays the **four Fs: fat, female, forty, and fertile**. The disease also appears very frequently among Pima Indians and has an increased incidence among African Americans.

Management **Surgical intervention** is often recommended in cases where symptoms began within 72 hours of presentation. Among patients who present later and who respond to medical therapy (NPO, NG tube, IV fluids, and antibiotics), cholecystectomy should be scheduled for 4 to 6 weeks later. If conservative therapy fails, if there is any suspicion of an empyema or perforation, or if acalculous cholecystitis is suspected, emergent cholecystectomy is indicated. **ERCP** may be used to remove common bile duct stones; **cholecystostomy** (percutaneous drainage) may be attempted in high-risk surgical candidates. Gangrenous cholecystitis in elderly patients and diabetics may have a benign presentation.

Complications **Ascending cholangitis** should be suspected in the presence of **Charcot's triad** (fever, pain, and jaundice) or **Reynold's pentad** (Charcot's triad plus shock and mental status alteration).

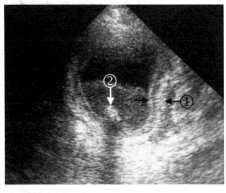

[A]

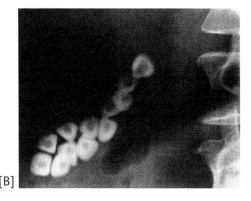

[B]

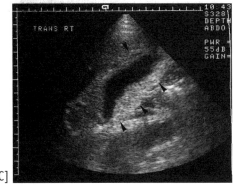

[C]

Gallbladder empyema, gallbladder perforation, gallstone pancreatitis, pericholecystic abscess, and cholecystenteric fistulas are other potential complications.

Atlas Link   ⬛⬛⬛⬛ PG-P2-002

MINICASE 343: CHOLANGIOCARCINOMA

Adenocarcinoma of intra- or extrahepatic bile ducts
- associated with chronic cholecystitis or infection by *Clonorchis sinensis*
- presents with pruritus, jaundice, dark urine, clay-colored stool (due to obstructive jaundice), and a palpable gallbladder
- treat with stenting to temporarily open bile ducts and alleviate symptoms
- the tumor invariably causes death within 1 to 2 years

MINICASE 344: CHOLEDOCHOLITHIASIS

Gallstones in bile ducts seen most commonly in middle-aged, obese, multiparous females or patients with chronic hemolysis
- presents with intermittent biliary colic, fever, and jaundice (CHARCOT'S TRIAD)
- US demonstrates dilated bile duct, ERCP demonstrates the presence of obstructing gallstones
- treatment is ERCP-guided removal of obstructing gallstones, sphincterotomy of the ampulla of Vater, and laparoscopic cholecystectomy
- complications include ascending cholangitis, hepatic abscesses, and sepsis

---

MINICASE 345: CHOLELITHIASIS

Gallstones in the gallbladder, most commonly seen in females who are fat, fertile, and over 40 (four Fs) or in chronic hemolytic states
- uncomplicated cholelithiasis may be asymptomatic or may present with dyspepsia and intolerance to fatty foods
- the clinical picture may be complicated by acute cholecystitis or choledocholithiasis
- US reveals gallstones
- treat with cholecystectomy if symptomatic, otherwise no treatment is required

GENERAL SURGERY

ID/CC A 40-year-old obese male complains of **acute burning and tearing rectal pain** that began 2 hours ago with passage of a **very hard stool**.

HPI He states that he noticed **blood** on the toilet paper after the bowel movement and adds that he suffers from chronic **constipation**.

PE VS: normal. PE: unable to find a comfortable position to sit; anorectal exam reveals **sphincter spasm; linear ulceration of the anal mucosa** in posterior midline; **sentinel tag at distal margin of fissure** and **hypertrophic papilla proximal to fissure**.

Pathogenesis An anal fissure is a **linear tear in the anorectal mucosa** that is generally caused by **trauma** (from constipation, straining at stool, chronic diarrhea). Other causes include surgical operations in the anorectal area, cathartic abuse, chronic anxiety with spasm of the sphincter, Crohn's disease, ulcerative colitis, anal intercourse, syphilis, tuberculosis, and malignancy. Anal fissures may be acute or chronic, and the patient characteristically complains of **minimal bleeding** and **severe pain during stool passage** that may last from minutes to several hours. Chronic fissures present similarly with anal **ulcers, a sentinel pile** (a pouch of skin at the anal verge), and **hypertropic papillae** on exam.

Epidemiology Anal fissures occur primarily in young and middle-aged adults and show no gender predominance. An increased incidence is seen with receptive anal intercourse and Crohn's disease. The condition may also coexist with hemorrhoids and other colorectal diseases.

Management The vast majority of simple cases respond to medical therapy with **stool softeners, high-fiber diet, analgesics, sitz baths**, and **anesthetic suppositories**. Topical nitrates and botulinum toxin have met with some success. In chronic, refractory cases, **lateral internal sphincterotomy** may be performed. The fissure itself as well as the pile and papillae may also be resected. If the fissure is not acute, **sigmoidoscopy** (to evaluate for Crohn's disease) should be done to assess the distal colon and rectum. Nonhealing ulcers should be biopsied to rule out cancer.

Complications   Chronicity, recurrence, infection, abscess formation, fistulas, contact dermatitis to local anesthetic agents and ointments, postoperative bleeding, urinary retention, chronic mucus discharge, and fecal incontinence (mostly to liquid stool and gas).

Atlas Link   UCV2   SUR-018

MINICASE 346: CYSTIC HYGROMA

A benign neoplasm of the lymphatic vessels most commonly found in the posterior triangle of the neck in infants and in the mediastinum or retroperitoneum in adults
- presents at birth or in infancy with considerable neck enlargement, occasionally complicating delivery, and with problems swallowing and breathing
- mass can usually be transilluminated
- treat surgically, although complete removal is difficult in that the lesion tends to grow into vital neck structures

MINICASE 347: DECUBITUS ULCER

Ischemic tissue necrosis and skin ulceration caused by prolonged pressure, most frequently at bony prominences
- presents in immobile or bedridden patients with skin breakdown over the sacrum, trochanter, ankles, and heels
- treat by avoiding prolonged pressure, frequent turning, use of air mattresses, good nutrition, antibiotics for infection, surgery for deep ulcers

MINICASE 348: EPISPADIAS

A rare congenital anomaly in which the urethral meatus is located on the dorsal aspect of the penis
- almost always associated with bladder exstrophy
- presents with marked dorsiflexion of the penis and urinary incontinence (commonly seen in the penopubic and penile types, uncommonly with the glandular type)
- treat with surgical correction of the penile curvature, urethral reconstruction, and bladder-neck reconstruction in incontinent patients

ID/CC A 49-year-old **man** presents with **intermittent, foul-smelling, purulent anal discharge** that stains his underwear.

HPI The discharge is occasionally accompanied by itching.

PE PE: posterior **opening in the perianal skin** through which a purulent exudate and stool are digitally expressed; irritation of skin surrounding opening; fistulous tract is firm and fibrotic; no fluctuation (sign of abscess) noted.

Labs CBC: mild leukocytosis ($13,500/mm^3$).

Pathogenesis An anal fistula is a **fibrous communication between an anal crypt and the perianal skin**. It is usually **secondary to a previous anorectal abscess**, with its origin in Morgagni's crypts. Crohn's disease, tuberculosis, trauma, radiation, lymphogranuloma venereum, diverticulitis, and anorectal neoplasia may also cause a fistula. Fistulas may be multiple. **Goodsall's rule** states that fistulas that drain through an opening posterior to a transverse line through the anus (looking at the supine patient from the feet) originate from a posterior midline crypt and take a curved path; anterior fistulas drain anterior crypts and take a straight path.

Epidemiology Seen predominantly in **males**; most fistulas drain a septic-purulent cavity (ANORECTAL ABSCESS). Fecal incontinence of varying degrees can occur. Also associated with Crohn's disease.

Management **Rectosigmoidoscopy** must be performed in all cases prior to surgery to assess the terminal colon and rectum. Generally a **barium enema** is also done. **Fistulography** with contrast media may help delineate complex fistulas. Surgery is nearly always indicated due to scarring and chronicity. A **fistulotomy** involves "unroofing" the fistulous tract with marsupialization of borders; **fistulectomy** involves excision of the tract with the surrounding fibrous tissue. A seton (a suture run through the fistulous tract that is progressively tightened to induce fibrosis) may be used in some patients. Contraindications to surgery include inflammatory bowel disease and HIV infection.

Complications Chronicity; spread of infection; malignant degeneration; and puborectalis muscle injury during surgery, leading to incontinence.

ID/CC	A 15-year-old boy presents with **severe right lower quadrant pain**.
HPI	He states that he began to experience abdominal pain near the **umbilicus** (referred pain from sympathetic fibers) yesterday. It gradually worsened and was followed by nausea and vomiting, **loss of appetite** (ANOREXIA), and difficulty defecating. As the pain worsened, it became sharp and migrated to **McBurney's point** (one-third of the distance from the anterior superior iliac spine to the umbilicus).
PE	VS: **tachycardia** (HR 108); normal BP; low-grade fever (38.2°C). PE: abdomen tense with diminished bowel sounds; exquisite tenderness over **McBurney's point; rebound tenderness** localizing to right lower quadrant; pain on passive extension of hip while lying on left side with knee extended (PSOAS SIGN); pain on passive internal rotation of hip (INTERNAL OBTURATOR SIGN); right lower quadrant tenderness with deep palpation of left lower quadrant (ROVSING'S SIGN); right side of rectovesical pouch tender on rectal exam.
Labs	CBC: **leukocytosis** (14,300/mm^3) with **neutrophilia**. UA: normal (mild pyuria and hematuria are not uncommon).
Imaging	CXR: normal. KUB: radiopaque **fecalith** in appendicular area (rare); localized **ileus** in the right lower quadrant with air-fluid levels. US, **[A]** longitudinal and **[B]** transverse: noncompressible, dilated, tubular appendix with edematous wall (double-headed arrows). **[C]** CT, abdomen: inflammatory pericecal mass in the right iliac fossa.
Pathogenesis	Appendicitis occurs following **obstruction of the appendiceal lumen** as a result of lymphoid hyperplasia, a fecalith, a foreign body, a parasitic infection (ascariasis, amebiasis, trichuriasis), or a stricture. Mucus is secreted into the obstructed lumen, providing a good medium for bacterial growth and inflammation. Additionally, increased luminal and wall pressure leads to ischemia, infarction, and necrosis of the appendix. The appendix may subsequently perforate, causing diffuse peritonitis and sepsis, or it may form an abscess. The appendix may be retrocecal (causing maximal pain in the right lateral, pelvic, or paracolic regions).
Epidemiology	Acute appendicitis is one of the most common surgical conditions; a diet high in refined sugars and meat is a predisposing factor. The incidence is lower in developing countries. Young

GENERAL SURGERY

APPENDICITIS—ACUTE

patients develop the condition more frequently. Elderly patients may not present with the same signs and symptoms as the young (in such patients, appendicitis may present only as hypotension).

Management **No analgesics or antibiotics** should be administered until a final diagnosis or a decision to operate has been made (withholding analgesics is controversial). **Emergent appendectomy**. Administer postoperative antibiotics that cover gram-positive, gram-negative, and anaerobic organisms (ampicillin + gentamicin + metronidazole). Localized, walled-off abscesses may be treated first with ultrasound-guided or **[D] CT-guided percutaneous drainage** followed by interval or delayed appendectomy 2 to 4 weeks later.

Complications Complications include pylephlebitis, appendiceal abscess, peritonitis, appendiceal perforation, residual (subphrenic, pelvic) or wall sepsis, and fistula. An incidental carcinoid is found in 1 in 250 appendectomies.

Atlas Links ⬚⬚⬚⬚ PG-P2-003, PM-P2-003

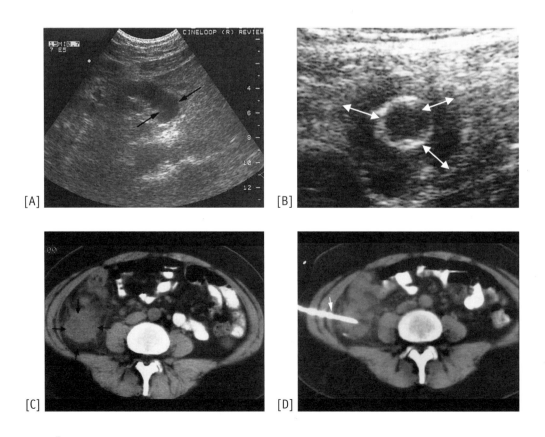

[A] [B] [C] [D]

ID/CC	A 67-year-old man presents with an unexplained 10-kg **weight loss** over the past 6 months.
HPI	His bowel habits have changed recently with **alternating diarrhea** and **constipation, decreased stool caliber**, and occasional passage of bright red blood mixed with stool (HEMATOCHEZIA).
PE	VS: normal. PE: thin; mild scleral icterus; abdomen soft and nontender; mild **hepatomegaly** (due to metastases); rectal exam reveals large, nontender, **hard mass 5 cm from anal verge**; bright red blood on examining finger.
Labs	CBC: anemia. LFTs: **increased alkaline phosphatase** (due to hepatic metastases). **Increased CEA** (not specific for colon cancer; also increased with hepatocellular carcinoma).
Imaging	**[A]** BE: the classic **"apple core" filling defect** is seen in the sigmoid colon. **[B]** BE: a different case demonstrates a sessile polypoid lesion in the sigmoid colon. **[C]** CT, abdomen: after insufflation of air into the colon, a sessile polypoid lesion is seen in another patient. **[D]** CT, pelvis: another case shows tumor invasion into the peripelvic fat and bladder (B) wall.
Pathogenesis	More than 95% of colorectal cancers **progress from a benign neoplastic polyp** to a malignant neoplasm. Defects in p53, *ras,* and APC, as well as a number of other genetic mutations, have been well described. **Polyps > 1 cm, those with villous morphology, and those with severe atypia are most likely to be malignant**. Colon cancer is associated with **diets high in refined carbohydrates and animal fat and low in fiber**. Dietary carcinogens, bile salts, and slow bowel-content transit time produce changes in the mucosa that predispose to cancer in **genetically susceptible individuals**. The most common anatomic location is the **rectum/sigmoid**; the most common type is **adenocarcinoma**. While **left-sided** tumors **spread circumferentially** and manifest with an early decrease in **stool caliber** and a change in bowel habits along with **obstructive symptoms**, early **right-sided** cancer may be asymptomatic except for **constitutional symptoms** such as fatigue, weight loss and **anemia**, or melena from occult bleeding. Rectal lesions are also associated with tenesmus and may cause frank rectal bleeding.
Epidemiology	Colon cancer is the most common visceral cancer and the **third most common form of cancer** in the United States, affecting men and women equally. A higher incidence is reported in Western countries (most likely secondary to dietary patterns). The risk of malignant degeneration in patients with **familial adenomatous**

polyposis and **Gardner's syndrome** (osteomas of the skull, colonic polyps, and skin tumors) is 100%. Patients with **Turcot's syndrome** (colonic polyposis and CNS tumors), breast cancer, chronic ulcerative colitis, and Crohn's disease, as well as those with a **family history** of colon cancer in a first-degree relative, are at increased risk.

Management **Surgery** consists of right or left colectomy with lymph node resection depending on the location, with primary anastomosis or generation of an ostomy. Pre- or postoperative chemotherapy and radiotherapy may be given to prevent recurrences or for inoperable tumor palliation. **Dukes** staging (based on extension through the bowel wall) is the best predictor of recurrences and mortality; lung and hepatic metastases worsen the prognosis. Sigmoidoscopy every 3 to 5 years in patients older than 50 and yearly occult blood and yearly digital rectal exam for patients younger than 40 are recommended for prevention.

Complications Metastatic disease, bowel obstruction, bowel perforation, abdominal fistulas, and urinary tract obstruction.

Atlas Link   UCV2 **SUR-021**

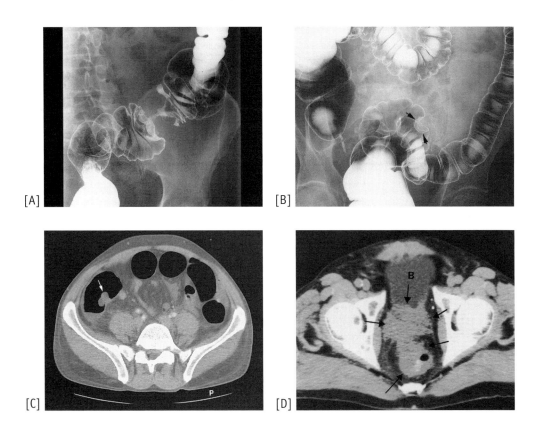

[A]   [B]   [C]   [D]

ID/CC A **75-year-old black man** presents with lack of appetite (ANOREXIA) and progressive **difficulty swallowing** (DYSPHAGIA), starting with **solids** and then progressing to **liquids**.

HPI He also reports **painful swallowing** (ODYNOPHAGIA) and a 7-kg weight loss. He **smokes** two packs of cigarettes per day and acknowledges heavy **alcohol** intake. Directed questioning reveals occasional vomiting and regurgitation.

PE VS: normal. PE: **emaciated** with **pallor**; vocal cords mobile bilaterally; cervical adenopathy; **fixed, palpable, nontender left supraclavicular lymph node** (VIRCHOW'S NODE).

Labs CBC: **decreased hemoglobin** (8.4 gm/dL) (anemia from occult bleeding); decreased WBC count. ESR mildly elevated; **hypercalcemia; hypoalbuminemia.** LFTs: increased AST and ALT (hepatic metastases). **Heme-positive stool**; endoscopy reveals obstructing, irregular, polypoid, exophytic mass; biopsy shows **squamous cell carcinoma**.

Imaging **[A]** UGI: proximal dilatation with **filling defect** in the middle third of the esophagus. **[B]** UGI: a different case revealing an extensive **exophytic mass** in the middle third of the esophagus. **[C]** CT, chest: another case showing a mass (1) surrounding the esophageal lumen (2) and invading the mediastinum; an enlarged subcarinal lymph node (N) is also shown. CT, abdomen: numerous hepatic metastases.

Pathogenesis Esophageal carcinoma is associated with **alcohol** abuse, **cigarette** smoking, achalasia, irradiation to the chest, **chronic esophagitis**, nitrosamines, leukoplakia, Plummer–Vinson syndrome, exposure to aniline dyes, stricture from caustic ingestion (lye strictures), gastroesophageal reflux disease, and **Barrett's esophagus** (glandular metaplasia of the distal esophagus caused by chronic gastroesophageal reflux). The most common type is **squamous cell** (EPIDERMOID), and the most common site is the **upper two-thirds** of the esophagus. The lower third of the esophagus is more commonly associated with **adenocarcinoma** arising from Barrett's esophagus. PE is often unremarkable apart from emaciation. Tumors frequently spread locally (the esophagus is without a serosal layer) by direct extension and via lymphatics; distant metastases are to the liver, lung, bone, and adrenals. The mass is **initially painless**, but mediastinal spread may cause **chest pain**, and laryngeal nerve involvement may cause **hoarseness**. Phrenic nerve involvement may cause respiratory distress.

ESOPHAGEAL CARCINOMA

Epidemiology   Esophageal carcinoma occurs in 5 in 100,000 people in the United States and has a predilection for **older men**. Additionally, there has been a striking increase in the squamous cell type among African Americans. The incidence of adenocarcinoma is also increasing markedly (due to Barrett's). The prognosis is poor; the overall **5-year survival rate is 5%**.

Management   Endoscopy with **multiple biopsies** (submucosal spread may yield false negatives) is necessary for accurate diagnosis. In high-risk populations, **periodic endoscopy** is needed for early detection (representing the only chance for cure). If cure is possible, then **surgical resection** with **preoperative chemotherapy** and **radiotherapy** is preferred. **Palliative radiotherapy, chemotherapy,** endoscopic laser, or stent placement is offered for patients with metastasis or significant local spread and for poor surgical candidates.

Complications   Metastatic disease, occult bleeding, tracheal obstruction, tracheo- and bronchoesophageal fistula, and aspiration pneumonia.

Atlas Links   ⬚⬚⬚⬚⬚ PG-P2-005A, PG-P2-005B

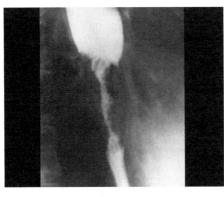

[A]

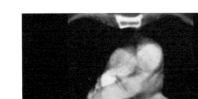

[C]

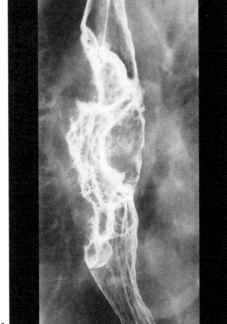

[B]

ID/CC A 51-year-old **female** presents with **sudden** onset of **pain** in her right **groin** with a **tense and tender mass** in the region.

HPI She **was carrying a heavy box** when the pain began. Several months ago she noticed a mass in the right groin that was small and nonpainful and that protruded with exercise, but the mass disappeared spontaneously.

PE VS: **tachycardia**; normal BP; **fever** (38.1°C). PE: **abdomen slightly distended, tympanic** (intestine is obstructed with backward accumulation of gas and feces), and tender to palpation; tense, acutely tender, 1.5-cm mass in right groin with changes in skin color below inguinal ligament; mass **does not reduce with pressure**.

Labs CBC: **leukocytosis with neutrophilia**.

Imaging **[A]** XR, abdomen: a Gastrografin follow-through study shows **dilated loops of small bowel** secondary to obstruction by an incarcerated right femoral hernia.

Pathogenesis A hernia **strangulation** occurs when the constricting hernial ring compromises the blood supply, resulting in **ischemia and**

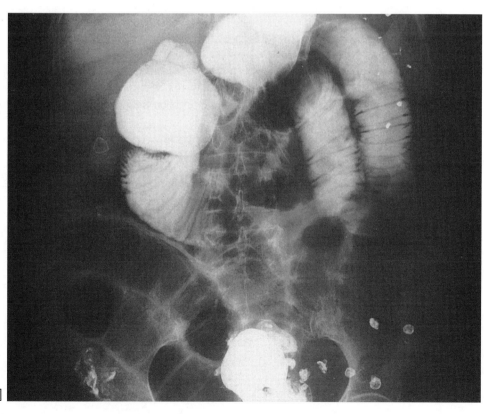

[A]

STRANGULATED FEMORAL HERNIA

necrosis; this process may lead to **perforation**. The incidence of all hernias and associated strangulation increases with any factor that **increases intra-abdominal pressure**, including obesity, chronic cough, lifting heavy objects, and straining at stool or micturition.

Epidemiology **Femoral hernias strangulate more commonly** than inguinal or umbilical hernias. Inguinal hernias are more common in males, while **femoral hernias are more common in females**.

Management **Emergent surgery** after the patient is stabilized with aggressive IV resuscitation. Antibiotics are usually administered. Bowel resection is performed if a segment of nonviable intestine is found.

Complications May be associated with infection, abscess, hematoma and granuloma formation, damage to the ilioinguinal nerve, and recurrence. Strangulation may lead to **perforation** with generalized **peritonitis**, intra-abdominal abscess formation, or sepsis. The femoral hernial sac is in close proximity to the **femoral vein**, which may be damaged during surgery.

MINICASE 349: HEMANGIOMA

A benign neoplasm of endothelium that commonly regresses during childhood
- may be associated with other systemic congenital disorders
- presents with an erythematous, vascular-appearing growth that can be raised or flat
- treat with laser coagulation, although in children many lesions regress spontaneously
- complications include scarring

Atlas Links: U C V 2 MC-349A, MC-349B, MC-349C

MINICASE 350: HEMORRHOIDS—EXTERNAL

Dilatation of the veins of the inferior hemorrhoidal plexus
- presents with rectal bleeding, becoming painful if thrombosed
- treat with high-fiber diet, sitz baths
- if severe or refractory, consider rubber band ligation or hemorrhoidectomy

ID/CC   A **71-year-old female** nursing-home resident presents with abdominal pain, **nausea, vomiting**, and **inability to pass flatus and stool** (OBSTIPATION) for 3 days.

HPI   For the past 3 years she has been having **episodes of "stomach upset"** (biliary colic due to cholelithiasis) that she treats with OTC antacids. She has no history of prior surgery.

PE   VS: **tachycardia** (HR 101); low-grade fever (38.1°C). PE: dry oropharynx (due to dehydration from intraluminal third spacing); **abdomen distended, tympanitic, and tender** in all four quadrants; no rebound tenderness; increased bowel sounds; rectal exam unremarkable.

Labs   CBC: **moderate leukocytosis with left shift**. LFTs: normal. ABGs: **metabolic alkalosis** (due to vomiting). Lytes: low potassium and chloride.

Imaging   **[A]** SBFT: dilated loops of jejunum are seen along with a filling defect that represents the **gallstone**. **[B]** SBFT: a different case that again demonstrates dilated loops of small bowel and a distal filling defect representing a gallstone. **[C]** SBFT: another case showing a **round opacity in the pelvis** that was found to be a gallstone at the time of operation (only 15% of gallstones are radiopaque). XR, abdomen: demonstrates **gas in the biliary tree** (PNEUMOBILIA) secondary to a cholecystenteric fistula.

Pathogenesis   Gallstone ileus results from intestinal obstruction at the level of the ileocecal valve (narrowest portion of small intestine). **Stones formed in the gallbladder gain access to the intestine through a pathologic communication** (FISTULA) between the gallbladder and the intestine (usually the duodenum). These arise as a result of recurrent attacks of gallbladder inflammation with adhesions and scarring. Stones may also pass into the peritoneal cavity, causing extraluminal inflammation and obstruction. Stones that are passed to the GI tract through the biliary ducts are too small to block the ileocecal valve and therefore do not cause gallstone ileus.

Epidemiology   Gallstone ileus is a disease of the **elderly**. There is frequently a delay in diagnosis. Gallstone ileus carries a substantial mortality rate.

GALLSTONE ILEUS

Management	**Emergent laparotomy** with **enterotomy** to extract the stone. Concurrent cholecystectomy and fistula closure may be performed. Palpate to rule out the presence of additional stones prior to closure.
Complications	Recurrence in 10% of cases, perforation, and sepsis.

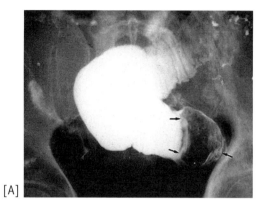

[A]

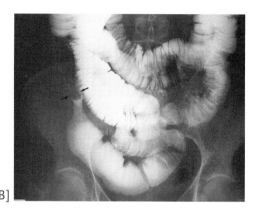

[B]

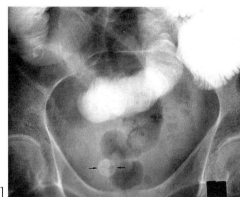

[C]

ID/CC	A 69-year-old **Japanese man** complains of **loss of appetite** and an 11-kg **weight loss** over 9 months.
HPI	He is a former **smoker** (quit 5 years ago), has **group A+** blood, and suffers from arthritis. He has a history of *Helicobacter pylori* infection and **gastric ulcers**. His father died of stomach cancer.
PE	VS: normal. PE: pallor; **muscle wasting**; nontender **left supraclavicular lymphadenopathy** (VIRCHOW'S SENTINEL NODE); left axillary lymphadenopathy; abdomen flat with scant adipose pad; mild **hepatomegaly** (metastases); nontender umbilical nodule (SISTER MARY JOSEPH'S NODULE); mild **ascites**.
Labs	CBC: **anemia** (Hb 7.6 gm/dL). **Hypoalbuminemia**; increased CEA (not specific); stool **heme positive**. LFTs: elevated AST and ALT; elevated alkaline phosphatase (hepatic metastases).
Imaging	**[A]** UGI: marked loss of distensibility of the antrum due to narrowing and circumferential mass (1). **[B]** CT, abdomen (with oral contrast): the lumen of the stomach is filled with white contrast, revealing a large, ulcerated soft tissue mass (1) on the lesser curvature. There is also evidence of celiac lymph node involvement (2) and hepatic metastases (3). **[C]** UGI: a different case demonstrates a malignant ulcer; the mucosal folds do not reach the ulcer crater (unlike benign ulcers).
Pathogenesis	Risk factors and causative associations include **chronic *H. pylori* infection** (for distal tumors), **hypertrophic gastritis** (MÉNÉTRIER'S DISEASE), **chronic atrophic gastritis** with intestinal metaplasia, **pernicious anemia**, partial gastrectomy (usually Billroth II), a family history of gastric cancer in a first-degree relative, and diets low in vegetables/fruits and high in **nitrosamines, smoked fish**, and heavily salted foods. Morphologic types include **ulcerative, polypoid**, superficially spreading (best prognosis), and **diffusely infiltrative** (**linitis plastica**; worst prognosis). **Dyspeptic symptoms** or **skin manifestations** (acanthosis nigricans) may be the only initial complaints. The location and type of tumor determine the nature of the symptoms: vomiting (pylorus), dysphagia (cardia), weight loss (linitis), and bleeding (ulcerative). The disease yields deceptively **few symptoms until it is advanced**, especially linitis plastica. Antral tumors are the most common; local invasion is more common than metastasis. The prognosis is generally poor; only 40% of patients have resectable disease at presentation.

GASTRIC CARCINOMA

Epidemiology   Incidence increases with age and is rare before age 40. There is a high incidence in Japan (80 times higher than in the United States), Chile, and Central America as well as among African Americans, Asians, and Hispanics. A 2-to-1 male predominance has been noted.

Management   **Surgical resection** (total or subtotal gastrectomy) represents the only chance for cure, although only a small percentage of cases are operable. CT, MR, and endoscopy may determine resectability, but only laparotomy can do so with certainty. **Total parenteral nutrition** is often used preoperatively due to cachexia. Lymph node dissection, splenectomy, or omentectomy may be necessary. Chemotherapy and radiotherapy have proven ineffective. **Palliative resection** or bypass with gastrojejunostomy improves the quality of life.

Complications   Fistula to colon, obstruction, bleeding and perforation, and metastatic disease.

Atlas Link   UCV1 PG-P2-006

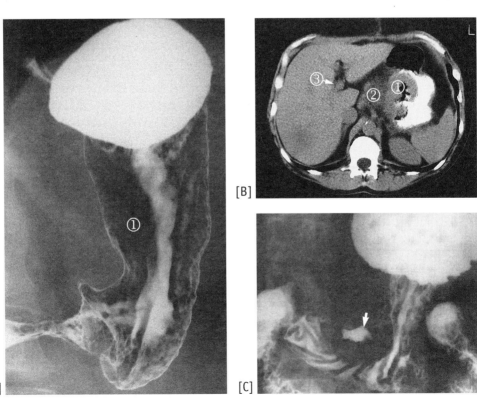

[A]

[B]

[C]

ID/CC	A 58-year-old man presents to the ER after passing a large amount of bright red blood per rectum (HEMATOCHEZIA).
HPI	He reports that he has always eaten a **low-fiber diet** and suffers from **chronic constipation**.
PE	VS: mild tachycardia; mild hypotension. PE: no acute distress; abdomen soft; **mild tenderness in left lower quadrant** with no masses; no hepatosplenomegaly or ascites; no peritoneal signs; rectal exam reveals frank bright blood in rectal vault; no hemorrhoids.
Labs	CBC/Lytes: normal. PT and PTT normal; colonoscopy reveals multiple **diverticula** of left colon; active bleeding from the neck of one.
Imaging	**[A]** BE: diverticular disease of the colon in the sigmoid colon (common location due to high intraluminal pressure). **[B]** A different case with diverticular disease of the ascending colon and appendix.
Pathogenesis	Lower GI bleeding occurs distal to the ligament of Treitz. It is associated with **diverticulosis, AV malformations**, ischemic bowel disease, colon cancer, polyposis, **hemorrhoids**, fissures, radiation colitis, inflammatory bowel disease (Crohn's, ulcerative colitis), Meckel's diverticula (ectopic gastric mucosa), and telangiectasias (Osler–Rendu–Weber's). Very brisk bleeds regardless of site and bleeding from very distal sites produce hematochezia, whereas slow, proximal bleeds produce melena, since stool color relates to time spent in the gut.
Epidemiology	Lower GI bleeds occur most commonly in the **elderly**. With severe bleeds, the mortality rate is approximately 10%. Diverticulosis, the most common cause of lower GI bleeding in adults, is associated with a low-fiber diet. There is an increased incidence of diverticular disease in patients with connective tissue disorders (e.g., Marfan's syndrome, Ehlers–Danlos syndrome).

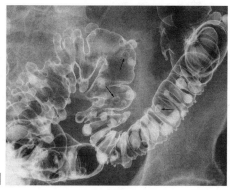

[A]

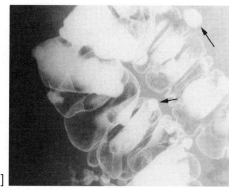

[B]

GASTROINTESTINAL BLEEDING—LOWER

Management   Hemodynamic stabilization and resuscitation, including packed RBCs or fresh frozen plasma for coagulation defects. An **anorectal exam** should be performed to rule out hemorrhoids, anal fissures, and other anorectal pathology. Next, an upper GI bleed should be ruled out by passing a **nasogastric tube** to look for blood. If there is evidence of blood, an EGD should be performed. With evidence of bile but no blood in the nasogastric tube, **anoscopy** and/or **sigmoidoscopy** should be performed. With slow bleeds, **colonoscopy** with or without subsequent tagged red cell scans (sensitive for slow bleeds > 0.1 cc/min) is usually adequate to establish a diagnosis. Massive bleeds will preclude diagnosis by colonoscopy, so an **angiogram** (sensitive to bleeds > 0.5 cc/min) is indicated. **Surgery** is recommended if bleeding is unresponsive to medical treatment or if the patient rebleeds. An exploratory laparotomy with endoscopy and a colectomy may be necessary if the source of bleeding cannot be determined. **Diverticulosis**: asymptomatic diverticulosis is managed with a **high-fiber diet**. Anticholinergics, antidepressants, and antibiotics have no proven effect.

Complications   Shock and death.

MINICASE 351: HEMORRHOIDS—INTERNAL

Varicosity of the internal hemorrhoidal plexus due to chronic constipation (straining during defecation) or portal hypertension
- presents with painless hematochezia
- hemorrhoids prolapsed through the rectum are visible, whereas nonprolapsed hemorrhoids are seen on proctoscopy
- treat with stool softeners and laxatives to relieve constipation, sitz baths for analgesia
- thrombosed hemorrhoids require excision

MINICASE 352: HYPOSPADIAS

The most common urethral congenital anomaly, characterized by a urethral meatus located on the ventral aspect of the penis
- takes several forms, including glandular, coronal, penoscrotal, and perineal
- presents with ventral curvature of the penis, difficulty controlling the urinary stream, ambiguous external genitalia, and a high incidence of cryptorchidism
- voiding cystourethrogram (VCUG) in severe anomalies, in the presence of genital ambiguity perform buccal smear and karyotype to establish genetic sex
- treat with surgical therapy before age 2

ID/CC	A **73-year-old** woman presents with a 3-day history of **dark, tarry stools** (MELENA).
HPI	She also reports **fatigue** and mild dizziness. She suffers from hypertension and rheumatoid arthritis, for which she takes **aspirin** daily.
PE	VS: **tachycardia** (HR 115); **orthostatic hypotension**. PE: pale; abdomen soft with mild generalized tenderness; no masses; no hepatomegaly or ascites.
Labs	CBC: **anemia** (Hb 7.8 gm/dL). **BUN increased**; nasogastric tube insertion reveals **"coffee-ground" blood** (blood changes color when exposed to hydrochloric acid); endoscopy shows diffuse erythema and multiple pinpoint **ulcerations** in gastric mucosa in fundus, body, and antrum with no active bleeding.
Imaging	**[A]** UGI: small punctate collections of barium surrounded by a halo that represents mucosal edema are seen in this patient with erosive gastritis. **[B]** UGI: a different case demonstrating similar lesions of erosive gastritis. **[C]** UGI: barium filling an ulcer crater in the duodenal bulb is seen in another patient.
Pathogenesis	A UGI bleed occurs proximal to the ligament of Treitz. **Duodenal ulcers** (40%) are the most common cause of UGI bleeds, but a variety of disease processes may be responsible, including **gastric ulcer, erosive gastritis** (hypertrophic, alcoholic, drug-induced [NSAIDs, steroids, aspirin]), **esophageal varices, Mallory–Weiss tears, and gastric cancer**. Other causes include aortoduodenal fistula, stress ulcers (Curling's in burns, trauma), hemobilia, duodenal diverticula, benign tumors, telangiectasia, and ruptured aneurysms of the GI tract. Chronic UGI bleeding is associated with iron deficiency anemia; acute UGI bleeding frequently presents with severe blood volume loss, a normal CBC, hypotension, tachycardia, low urine output, and shock.
Epidemiology	Annually, the incidence of hospitalization for UGI bleeding is approximately 15 in 10,000. **Elderly** patients are at especially high risk because of the prevalence of NSAID and aspirin use. UGI bleeds are more common in individuals with liver disease, diabetes, and coagulation disorders (such as advanced kidney disease).
Management	Patients should receive **two large-bore IVs** (routine labs, type and cross) and should be actively resuscitated with Ringer's and packed RBCs. A **nasogastric tube** should be inserted to

GASTROINTESTINAL BLEEDING—UPPER

determine the rate and amount of bleeding. Prior to the performance of an EGD, the patient should receive a **gastric lavage**. **Endoscopy** is useful both diagnostically and therapeutically (sclerotherapy, coagulation). **Surgery** is indicated if medical treatment fails. In **peptic ulcer disease**, if bleeding is active or if vessels are seen at the ulcer base, **endoscopic control** with epinephrine, polidocanol, cautery, and laser surgery may be attempted. Surgery for bleeding duodenal ulcers usually involves vagotomy and **pyloroplasty**; for severe gastric ulcers, a **gastrectomy** is sometimes performed. **Mallory–Weiss tears** spontaneously achieve hemostasis in 90% of cases. **Hemorrhagic gastritis** is treated with **ice lavage** and **angiographic vasopressin**. **Varices** require **sclerotherapy** or treatment with **octreotide** or **vasopressin** or transjugular intrahepatic portosystemic shunt (**TIPS**). In cases of hepatic failure, a surgical portosystemic shunt may be indicated.

Complications   Hemorrhagic shock, perforation, peritonitis, aspiration, and cardiac or cerebrovascular ischemia.

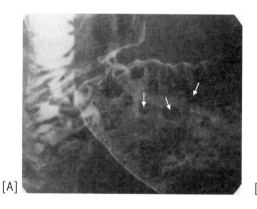

[A]

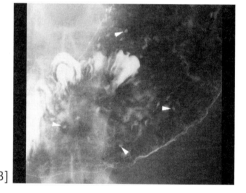

[B]

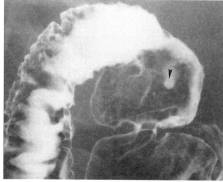

[C]

ID/CC A 27-year-old woman presents with an extremely tender **anal mass** associated with **acute perianal pain** and **bright red blood** during anal wiping.

HPI The patient is a **smoker** with a high stress level and a high-fat, **low-fiber diet**. She has a history of **chronic constipation**, anorectal pruritus, and grade II hemorrhoids (protrusion with defecation, spontaneous reduction).

PE VS: normal. PE: **[A]** rectal exam reveals a small, **well-defined, rounded, painful, purplish-red, firm mass** in anal margin with peripheral swelling (venous clot surrounded by inflammation).

Labs Proctoscopy: no rectal masses; grade II dilatation of internal hemorrhoidal venous plexus and thrombosed external hemorrhoid. (Note: in the presence of a thrombosed external hemorrhoid, proctoscopy is generally not performed.)

Pathogenesis Hemorrhoids are submucosal **venous dilatations** that may arise with increased **intra-abdominal pressure**, as occurs with straining on defecation or prolonged sitting or standing (associated with increased hydrostatic pressure). External hemorrhoids **arise distal to the dentate line** and may thrombose, causing acute pain and inflammation. These are often aggravated by consumption of spicy food, alcohol, chronic diarrhea, and anal infections. Internal hemorrhoids are generally painless.

Epidemiology Tumors, pregnancy, portal hypertension, chronic cough (COPD), prostatic hyperplasia, or straining at stool or urine may precipitate the onset and/or thrombosis of hemorrhoids.

Management Although most cases will **resolve spontaneously** within 2 weeks, **urgent hemorrhoidectomies** are generally recommended for

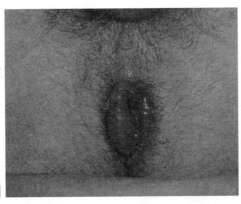

[A]

HEMORRHOIDS—INTERNAL-EXTERNAL

thrombosed external hemorrhoids in patients with severe pain. Patients who choose medical management over surgery should take warm **sitz baths** (thrice daily), receive **analgesics** and **stool softeners**, and **increase dietary fiber** intake. If medical treatment fails, symptoms recur, or complications arise (infection, bleeding), hemorrhoidectomy is again indicated.

Complications   Complications of surgery include incontinence, stricture formation, infections, and bleeding.

Atlas Link   U̲C̲V̲2̲ **SUR-028**

MINICASE 353: INTESTINAL MALROTATION WITH VOLVULUS

Congenital failure of the midgut to rotate properly during embryogenesis, allowing the small bowel to twist within the mesentery owing to lack of proper peritoneal attachment
- presents with bilious vomiting and abdominal distention
- AXR shows air-fluid levels and lack of gas in the colon
- CT or barium enema reveals the cecum lying outside the right lower quadrant
- treatment is emergent laparotomy with reduction of the volvulus and surgical correction of the malrotation

---

MINICASE 354: INTESTINAL PERFORATION

Rupture of internal viscera secondary to penetrating trauma, prolonged obstruction, or iatrogenic endoscopic manipulation
- presents with abdominal pain, rigidity with rebound tenderness, fever, and leukocytosis
- CXR or AXR shows intraperitoneal free air (PNEUMOPERITONEUM)
- treat with emergent laparotomy with repair of defect, ampicillin, gentamicin, and metronidazole
- complications include peritonitis and sepsis

MINICASE 355: KLATSKIN TUMOR

Carcinoma at the confluence of the extrahepatic bile ducts
- presents with cachexia, pruritus, nausea, vomiting, and jaundice
- may have right upper quadrant pain radiating to the back
- elevated alkaline phosphatase and conjugated hyperbilirubinemia
- treat with a stent at the duct confluence to palliate symptoms
- the tumor is relentlessly progressive

ID/CC	A 63-year-old construction worker complains of a **painful mass** in his **groin** that **enlarges with straining** and **disappears when he lies flat**.
HPI	The patient is a smoker with **emphysema** and **benign prostatic hypertrophy** (BPH).
PE	VS: normal. PE: barrel-shaped chest (due to COPD); abdomen soft, nontender, and nondistended; mass in inguinal region expands with coughing and diminishes with recumbency; when examining **finger is passed through scrotum into inguinal canal**, protrusion is felt on pad of finger (suggestive of direct inguinal hernia, whereas indirect hernias are felt on tip of finger).
Labs	Normal.
Imaging	**[A]** CT, abdomen: a different case with a small right inguinal hernia anterior to the common femoral artery.
Pathogenesis	A hernia is defined as a **protrusion of a viscus, or any part thereof**, through a **defect** in the **wall of the cavity** containing it. Inguinal hernias are classified as direct or indirect according to their anatomic relationship to the inferior epigastric vessels. **Indirect hernias** are due to **persistence of the processus vaginalis**. Herniation occurs **lateral** to the inferior epigastric artery, protrudes through the deep inguinal ring, and may extend into the scrotum. **Direct inguinal hernias** protrude through the floor of the inguinal canal (transversalis fascia and aponeurosis) through Hesselbach's triangle. These are associated with tissue laxity (as in old age) and with any factor that **increases intra-abdominal pressure**, such as obesity, chronic cough, or straining with bowel movements or micturition (e.g., BPH).

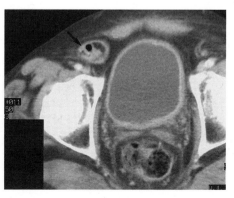

[A]

INGUINAL HERNIA

Epidemiology	Inguinal hernias account for 75% of all hernias, are more common in males (vs. femoral hernia), and are more commonly seen on the right side. **Indirect hernias are much more common** than direct hernias, particularly among children. Ten percent are bilateral.
Management	Acute incarceration or strangulation requires emergent surgical repair. In nonemergent cases, the patient is scheduled for **elective herniorrhaphy**.
Complications	**Incarceration** (irreducibility without vascular compromise), **strangulation** (ischemia and necrosis), perforated viscus, **intestinal obstruction** with fluid sequestration and electrolyte imbalance, and damage to the urinary bladder or spermatic cord during surgical repair.
Atlas Link	ⓊⒸⓋ② SUR-029

MINICASE 356: MESENTERIC ADENITIS

Painful enlargement of mesenteric lymph nodes caused by *Yersinia* spp, usually seen in children and young adults
- presents with right lower quadrant pain mimicking appendicitis, fever, and diarrhea
- stool shows *Yersinia enterocolitica* or *Y. pseudotuberculosis*
- diagnosis is made on laparotomy
- treat with fluoroquinolone

MINICASE 357: PAROTID GLAND—PLEOMORPHIC ADENOMA

The most common benign tumor of the salivary gland
- presents as a mass at the angle of the jaw, most commonly seen in middle-aged females
- histology shows uniform epithelial and myoepithelial cells distributed in cords, nests, and strands
- treat with wide local excision
- complications include high risk of recurrence and facial nerve damage

---

MINICASE 358: PERIANAL ABSCESS

Caused by infection in the perirectal spaces, most commonly polymicrobial infection due to *Escherichia coli*, *Proteus vulgaris*, streptococcus, staphylococcus, *Bacteroides*, and anaerobes
- presents with throbbing rectal pain, induration, erythema, warmth, and tenderness of the perirectal skin to palpation
- treat with incision and drainage
- complications include extension and fistula formation

ID/CC	A 40-year-old woman is admitted for several hours of **crampy abdominal pain, vomiting, abdominal distention**, and **inability to pass flatus or stool**.
HPI	She has had **multiple abdominal surgeries**, including an appendectomy, a total abdominal hysterectomy, a cholecystectomy, and, most recently, an incisional hernia repair.
PE	VS: **tachycardia** (HR 104); tachypnea; no fever. PE: **dry mucous membranes**; abdomen **tympanitic, distended**, and **tender** with no rigidity or rebound tenderness; **bowel sounds high-pitched and increased**; no stool in rectal vault.
Labs	CBC: **elevated hematocrit** (due to intraluminal fluid sequestration); elevated WBC count (16,400). Serum and urine amylase slightly increased (modest amylase elevations are seen in intestinal obstruction); lipase normal. ABGs: partially compensated metabolic **acidosis**.
Imaging	CXR: no free subdiaphragmatic air (no evidence of intestinal perforation); diminished excursion of the diaphragm (abdominal distention). **[A]** KUB: "string-of-beads" sign (1); no gas shadows in the colon or rectum (complete obstruction). **[B]** A different case with small bowel obstruction due to Crohn's disease demonstrating **dilated small bowel loops in a stepladder pattern** and **multiple air-fluid levels**.
Pathogenesis	**Mechanical obstruction** may be intrinsic (ascaris), extrinsic (hernia ring constricts bowel), or intramural (leiomyoma of wall blocks lumen). The **adynamic** (PARALYTIC) type involves no obstacle but is considered an obstruction because the end result is the same. Pressure increases proximal to the obstruction as fluid

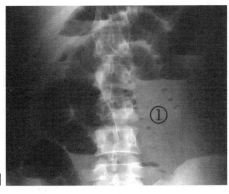

[A]

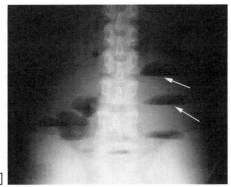

[B]

INTESTINAL OBSTRUCTION

and air build up. Over time, the pressure in the lumen may exceed the postcapillary venule pressure, impairing blood flow and eventually producing bowel ischemia and necrosis, leading to perforation. The most common causes of small bowel obstruction are **adhesions** (from prior surgery) and **hernias** (all types); other causes include **neoplasms** (in the elderly), **intussusception** (in infants), and parasites. Volvulus, usually of the cecum or sigmoid colon, causes large bowel obstruction with less prominent vomiting.

Epidemiology   Obstruction of the small bowel constitutes 75% of intestinal obstruction; obstruction of the colon constitutes 25%. In cases where the obstruction is relieved within 24 hours, mortality is only 1%. Otherwise, the obstruction can cause gangrene and perforation, leading to significant mortality.

Management   NPO; IV fluids; NG tube aspiration and decompression. Correction of fluid, electrolyte, and acid-base imbalances; broad-spectrum antibiotics; laparotomy with surgical resolution of obstruction.

Complications   Intestinal perforation, strangulation, peritonitis, recurrence of obstruction, systemic sepsis, and shock.

MINICASE 359: PETIT'S TRIANGLE HERNIA

Hernia arising from a triangle formed by the iliac crest, posterior border of the external oblique, and anterior border of the latissimus dorsi (PETIT'S TRIANGLE)
- affects all age groups, with males most frequently affected
- presents with a "lump near the buttocks" in the lumbar area and a rounded mass on exam
- treat with surgical repair

MINICASE 360: PILONIDAL CYST

A cyst in the sacrococcygeal area with associated granulation tissue, fibrosis, and hair tufts
- asymptomatic, but may become infected and present with pain, swelling, induration, and discharge from the skin in the midline sacrococcygeal area
- treat with incision and drainage, surgery for recurrent disease

ID/CC	A 23-year-old male student presents with prolonged high **fever with chills and diarrhea**.
HPI	Two weeks ago he underwent an appendectomy for **perforated appendicitis** with generalized peritonitis. He was discharged on antibiotics and had apparently recovered fully until the onset of his current symptoms.
PE	VS: **fever** (38.8°C); hypotension (BP 90/50); tachycardia (HR 105); normal RR. PE: **decreased breath sounds at right base**; abdomen soft with no rigidity; **tenderness to palpation in right upper quadrant**; surgical wound in right lower quadrant normal; no masses on rectal exam.
Labs	CBC: **elevated WBC** (16,700); 88% neutrophils with 12% bands.
Imaging	**[A]** CT, abdomen: a large abscess cavity with an air-fluid level (1) is seen between the right diaphragm and the right lobe of the liver. **[B]** CT, abdomen: a large retrocolic abscess (1) is seen in another patient with colon cancer (note the thickened wall of the colon). **[C]** XR, abdomen: a different case shows a large sub-phrenic abscess with an air-fluid level; the air on the left is the normal gastric bubble.
Pathogenesis	Most intra-abdominal abscesses result from **polymicrobial contamination** following surgery, usually by enteric gram-negative bacilli, gram-negative Enterobacteriaceae, or *Staphylococcus* and *Streptococcus*. Other causes include trauma; pyogenic infections such as appendicitis, diverticulitis, or cholecystitis; and hematogenous spread. An intra-abdominal abscess may present only with fever but may give rise to pain, sepsis, or diarrhea due to peritoneal irritation.
Epidemiology	Factors that **increase the risk of postoperative infection** include long hospital stays, anemia, malnourishment, the presence of hematomas or seromas, and emergency surgery that requires entry into unprepared bowel. The mortality rate of untreated abdominal abscesses approaches 100%.
Management	**Operative drainage** followed by broad-spectrum **antibiotics**. Ultrasound- or CT-guided **percutaneous drainage** is preferred for single, localized, accessible lesions.

31   **INTRA-ABDOMINAL ABSCESS**

Complications   Generalized peritonitis, systemic sepsis, wound dehiscence, and an increased incidence of postoperative hernias.

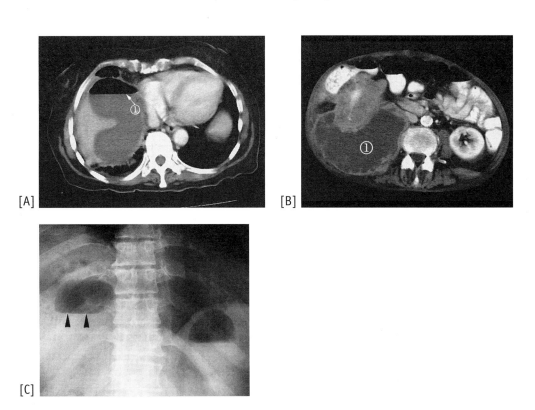

[A]

[B]

[C]

ID/CC   A **78-year-old** male nursing-home resident complains of dizziness, weakness, and acute-onset **severe, crampy abdominal pain**.

HPI   He adds that he **recently vomited** and had a **massive bowel movement**. He has had two **MIs** and underwent coronary artery bypass surgery (CABG); he is currently on digoxin for **atrial fibrillation and CHF**. He has **smoked** two packs of cigarettes a day for the past 30 years and also has **peripheral vascular disease** with **intermittent claudication**.

PE   VS: low-grade fever (38°C). PE: mildly **dehydrated**; diminished bowel sounds; **no rigidity or rebound tenderness**; abdomen slightly distended and extremely tender **(pain out of proportion to physical findings)**; **heme-positive stool**.

Labs   CBC: mild anemia (Hb 11.8 gm/dL); **marked leukocytosis** (20,050/mm^3) with **neutrophilia** (89% of total WBCs). Amylase moderately elevated.

Imaging   XR, abdomen: marked **distention of bowel loops with air-fluid levels; gas in bowel wall. BE: thumbprinting of mucosa.** Angio: vascular occlusion by embolus. **[A]** Angio: a different case demonstrating stenosis of the celiac artery (1) and inferior mesenteric artery (2) with a normal superior mesenteric artery (3).

Pathogenesis   Mesenteric ischemia may result from **thrombosis** (due to atherosclerotic vascular disease), **emboli** (due to **atrial fibrillation** or myocardial infarction), or **nonocclusive causes** (systemic arterial hypotension, prolonged CHF, dehydration). The ischemia usually results in life-threatening intestinal infarction. Because of collateral circulation, symptoms usually arise after compromise of two or more vessels. Other causes include portal hypertension, connective tissue disorders, vasculitis, hypercoagulable states (polycythemia

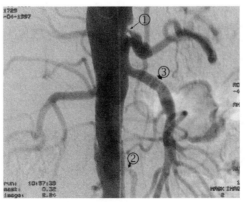

[A]

MESENTERIC ISCHEMIA

vera, protein C and S deficiency, antithrombin III deficiency), aneurysms, trauma, OCP use, and cocaine. Pain often fails to be alleviated even by strong analgesics, including narcotics.

Epidemiology   Mesenteric vascular disease occurs primarily in the **elderly** and is associated with extremely **high mortality** (approximately 80%). Other predisposing factors for vascular disease are hyperlipidemia, smoking, obesity, and diabetes mellitus.

Management   Patients with suspected mesenteric ischemia should receive aggressive volume resuscitation and broad-spectrum antibiotics. Laparotomy with **resection of necrotic bowel** is the mainstay of treatment. A "second look" laparotomy may be performed 24 hours later to ensure the viability of the remaining bowel. **Papaverine** is given if occlusion is seen on angiogram. **Interventional angiographic thrombolysis** can be performed for localized disease. **Thrombectomy** may be necessary.

Complications   Intestinal necrosis, perforation, generalized peritonitis, bacteremia, septic shock, ARDS, acute renal insufficiency, recurrence, short bowel syndrome, and the need for permanent total parenteral nutrition.

Atlas Link   ⬜C⬜⬜ PG-A-033

MINICASE 361: RICHTER'S HERNIA

Hernia in which only one wall of intestine is trapped by constricting ring of hernia
- more common in femoral hernia
- presents with a painful, tender groin mass
- bowel ischemia and necrosis occur with no signs of intestinal obstruction
- treat with immediate surgery to release ischemic-gangrenous bowel, hernia repair

---

MINICASE 362: SCOLIOSIS

Lateral curvature of the spine with associated rotation of the involved vertebrae
- asymptomatic in adolescence, more common in females
- S-shaped curvature is seen on forward flexion
- x-ray of the spine shows primary curvature
- curvatures < 20 degrees require no treatment, whereas those 20 to 40 degrees require bracing and those > 40 degrees require surgery
- complications include pulmonary compromise due to thoracic curvature

Atlas Links: ⬜C⬜⬜2 MC-362A, MC-362B

ID/CC   A **62-year-old man** is evaluated for **yellowing of the skin and weight loss**.

HPI   Directed questioning reveals **dark urine** (CHOLURIA) and **clay-colored stools** (ACHOLIA). He is a heavy **drinker** and **smoker**. He also complains of dull abdominal pain.

PE   VS: normal. PE: **emaciated** and markedly **jaundiced**; enlarged left supraclavicular lymph node (VIRCHOW'S NODE); nontender hepatomegaly (secondary to metastases); gallbladder is palpable and nontender (COURVOISIER'S SIGN); migratory thrombophlebitis (TROUSSEAU'S SYNDROME).

Labs   CBC: **low hemoglobin** (8.8 gm/dL). ESR moderately elevated; **elevated glucose** (245 mg/dL). LFTs: **markedly elevated alkaline phosphatase; elevated total bilirubin** (12 mg/dL); **mildly elevated transaminases**. Hypercalcemia; elevated CEA (not specific for pancreatic cancer); amylase and lipase moderately elevated; elevated **serum CA 19-9** levels (tumor marker for pancreatic cancer).

Imaging   **[A]** UGI: **displacement and narrowing of duodenal sweep** due to mass effect of the head of the pancreas with ragged edges of infiltration. **[B]** CT, abdomen: **heterogeneous mass** (1) **in the pancreatic head. [C]** CT, abdomen: a different case with a mass in the pancreatic tail. **[D]** CT, abdomen: another case with a mass in the pancreatic body (1) and multiple liver metastases (2).

Pathogenesis   The vast majority of pancreatic malignancies are **adenocarcinomas**, two-thirds of which are ductal in origin and arise in the pancreatic head. Pancreatic carcinoma has been associated with a mutation in the *K-ras* oncogene, Gardner's syndrome, and colonic polyposis. It is also associated with **diabetes mellitus** (the only cancer that is increased in diabetics), **chronic pancreatitis** (calcific), **cigarette smoking**, chronic gallbladder disease, previous gastrectomy, exposure to chemicals (β-naphthylamine, acetylaminofluorene, urea, nitrosamines, and benzidine), frequent consumption of grilled and fried red meat, and diets high in **fat, protein**, and **caffeine**. Metastatic disease (mesenteric and periaortic lymph nodes, peritoneum, liver, and lungs) is usually present at the time of diagnosis. The average survival after diagnosis is 9 months, and the 5-year survival rate is 5%.

PANCREATIC CARCINOMA

Epidemiology	More common among **elderly males**, blacks, Polynesians, and Native Americans, it is the fourth-leading cause of cancer death in the United States (approximately 25,000 per year). It generally presents between ages 50 and 70.
Management	If the cancer is resectable (no portal or superior mesenteric artery, liver, or hepatic artery involvement), a **pancreaticoduodenectomy** (WHIPPLE PROCEDURE) can be performed. Unresectable cases require **stenting, chemotherapy** or **radiation**, or bypass for palliation (e.g., cholecystojejunostomy). **Most cases are unresectable**.
Complications	**Portal vein thrombosis, gastric outlet obstruction, variceal bleeding**, metastatic disease, thromboembolic complications secondary to tumor-induced hypercoagulability, portal hypertension, splenomegaly, and jaundice.
Atlas Link	U C V 1 PG-P2-010

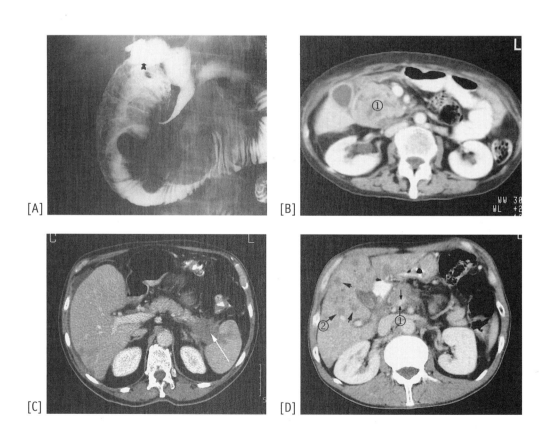

ID/CC	An 18-year-old male **motorcyclist** presents after colliding with an oncoming car; paramedics found him **unresponsive** and in **shock**.
HPI	After rapid infusion of 2 L of Ringer's, he regained consciousness and complained of **severe left-sided abdominal pain** with **left thoracic pain on inspiration**. The abdominal pain **radiated to the left scapula**.
PE	VS: no fever; **hypotension** (BP 80/40); **tachycardia** (HR 138). PE: alert and oriented; **skin cold and clammy** (hypovolemia); osseous crepitation (fracture) over left ribs 10 to 12; abdomen **distended**; guarding and left upper quadrant rebound tenderness; scapular pain on elevation of foot of bed or on palpation of left subcostal region (KEHR'S SIGN).
Labs	CBC: **anemia** (Hb 9.3 gm/dL); leukocytosis (16,300/mm^3) with 78% neutrophils. Four-quadrant peritoneal tap reveals **gross blood that does not coagulate**.
Imaging	CXR: elevation of the left hemidiaphragm; fracture of left ribs 10 to 12; no hemopneumothorax. US/CT: **hematoma surrounding the spleen** with obliteration of the splenic outline; free peritoneal fluid (blood).
Pathogenesis	**Blunt trauma** is the most common cause of splenic rupture. Since one-third of patients with a ruptured spleen do not initially present with frank hypotension and half may not have guarding and/or abdominal distention, a high index of suspicion must be maintained in all abdominal and chest trauma patients. Periodic clinical exams are needed to evaluate progress and surgical indications, as there may be a **latent period** between trauma and the onset of symptoms (BAUDET'S LATENT PERIOD).
Epidemiology	The spleen is the **most commonly injured intra-abdominal organ in blunt trauma. Lower rib fractures** are commonly associated with splenic rupture. Patients with **pathologic spleens** (due to hematologic disorders, infectious mononucleosis, malaria, leishmaniasis) are at higher risk.
Management	Follow **ATLS protocol for shock**: Airway, Breathing, Circulation, Disability, Exposure; place **two large-bore IVs**, place a Foley catheter, and perform abdominal paracentesis. Do not give pain

SPLENIC RUPTURE

medications until a therapeutic decision is made. A positive **diagnostic peritoneal lavage** has macroscopic blood $> 100,000$ RBCs/mm^3, > 500 WBCs/mm^3, bile, bacteria, or $> 1\%$ hematocrit in the aspirate. A **negative lavage does not exclude** visceral damage. **Immediate surgery** is indicated in the presence of a positive paracentesis, free intraperitoneal air, peritoneal signs, blood in the stomach or bladder, inability to resuscitate, penetrating wounds, or recurring signs of shock while under IV stabilization treatment. Postsplenectomy patients should receive prophylactic **pneumococcal and *Haemophilus influenzae* vaccinations. Grafting** may also be attempted (a portion of spleen should be left embedded in the omentum, which most likely will grow and, albeit partially, restore immunologic splenic function).

Complications   **Hemorrhagic shock, exsanguination**, atelectasis, postoperative subphrenic abscess or hematoma, and increased susceptibility to infections by encapsulated bacteria (e.g., *Meningococcus, Pneumococcus*). Postsplenectomy sepsis occurs only rarely after post-traumatic splenectomy.

Atlas Link   🅤🅒🅥🅘 PG-A-038

MINICASE 363: UMBILICAL HERNIA

Protrusion of the bowel through a congenital defect in the umbilical ring
- presents with an asymptomatic bulge through the umbilicus with increased abdominal pressure (e.g., lifting heavy weight)
- treatment is surgical reduction and repair of ring defect
- complications can include strangulation of bowel, leading to bowel necrosis

Atlas Links: 🅤🅒🅥🄲 MC-363A, MC-363B

MINICASE 364: VARICOSE VEINS

Dilatation and tortuosity of the superficial veins, most commonly in the lower extremities, caused by incompetence of valves or inherited weakness of the vessel wall
- commonly seen in obese, multiparous females
- presents with muscle fatigue, a feeling of heaviness in the lower extremities that worsens with prolonged standing, and dilated, elongated, and tortuous veins on the legs and thighs
- treat with weight loss, elastic stockings, avoidance of prolonged standing, surgery

Atlas Link: 🅤🅒🅥🄲 MC-364

ID/CC A **60-year-old man** complains of having **to wake up six to seven times at night to urinate** (NOCTURIA).

HPI He also complains of **urgency, weak stream, terminal dribbling**, and a need to strain in order to initiate micturition. The patient has had two episodes of **acute urinary retention** that required catheterization. He denies any weight loss, fatigue, or bone pain.

PE VS: normal. PE: cardiopulmonary and abdominal exams normal; rectal exam reveals **enlarged, nodular, nontender prostate** gland that is **rubbery** throughout and without a palpable median ridge; 150 cc of **residual urine** obtained on postvoid catheterization.

Labs UA: 8 WBCs per HPF; nitrates and leukocyte esterase positive; proteinuria and trace hematuria (due to concomitant infection). CBC: normal. Alkaline and acid phosphatase normal; PSA 5.5 (normal 5.4); BUN and creatinine normal; calcium normal.

Imaging US, prostate: enlarged prostate without focal mass; transrectal guided biopsy may be performed in multiple regions. **[A]** IVP:

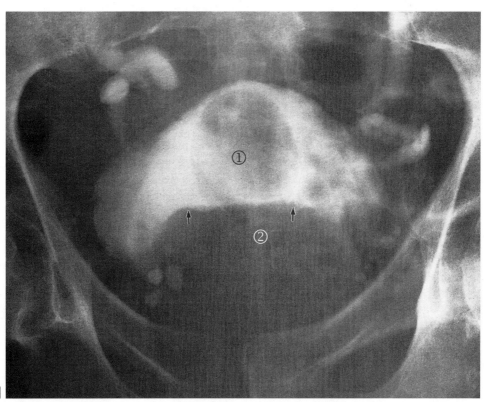

[A]

BENIGN PROSTATIC HYPERTROPHY (BPH)

another case reveals an elevated bladder (1) and an impression of the enlarged prostate (2) on the inferior surface.

Pathogenesis   Benign prostatic hypertrophy (BPH) occurs as a result of **hyperplasia of stromal and epithelial tissue** in the periurethral zone of aging men. This testosterone-dependent hyperplasia may cause **urinary flow obstruction and/or obstructive prostatism**. The size of the gland on physical exam generally does not correlate with symptoms. BPH usually originates in the periurethral and transition zones, while prostate cancer usually presents in the peripheral aspect of the prostate. It may coexist with carcinoma of the prostate, but **BPH is not considered a premalignant condition**. Note: cold exposure, anticholinergic drugs, anesthetic agents, and alcohol may precipitate or worsen symptoms.

Epidemiology   The **incidence of BPH increases with age**; $> 90\%$ of men have histologic evidence of BPH by age 85.

Management   Management is divided into medical and surgical therapies. Initial treatment is often medical with **5-α-reductase inhibitors** (e.g., finasteride) or **α-adrenergic blockers** (e.g., terazosin). **Surgery** may be done transurethrally (usually for glands < 50 g), or the traditional open prostatectomy (retropubic, suprapubic, or perineal approach) may be performed. Transurethral resection of the prostate **(TURP)** is the most common procedure, with newer procedures including transurethral balloon dilatation (TUBD) and transurethral incision of the prostate (TUIP; most useful for subtrigonal obstruction).

Complications   Complications include **urinary tract infections** (from stagnant urine), bladder diverticula, calculi, hydronephrosis, and chronic pyelonephritis. Common surgical complications are sexual **impotence** (especially with the transperineal approach) and **retrograde ejaculation**.

Atlas Link   ⬜UⒸⓋⓘ PG-P2-052

MINICASE 365: EPIDIDYMITIS

Painful inflammation of the epididymis caused by *Neisseria gonorrhoeae* and *Chlamydia trachomatis* in young men and by *Escherichia coli* and *Pseudomonas* in the elderly
• presents with unilateral scrotal edema and enlarged epididymis
• elevation of scrotal contents relieves pain (Prehn's sign)
• administer antibiotics

ID/CC A **70-year-old** man presents with **fresh blood in the urine** without pain (PAINLESS HEMATURIA).

HPI The patient has a 60-pack-year **smoking** history and has urinary **frequency** and **urgency**. He worked in an **aniline dye factory**.

PE VS: normal. PE: **pallor** (due to hematuria).

Labs CBC: anemia. Calcium and alkaline phosphatase normal. UA: 500 RBCs/HPF.

Imaging CXR: normal (rules out lung metastases). **[A]** IVP: large **filling defect** (1) in the left bladder with left ureter obstruction. **[B]** US, bladder: a different case with a large echogenic bladder tumor (1). **[C]** CT, bladder: another case with a focal tumor (T) on the bladder wall. Cystoscopy: 70% of lesions are **single** at the initial diagnosis.

Pathogenesis Although bladder cancer may be squamous, small cell, or adenocarcinoma, **> 90% are transitional cell in origin**. These tumors are generally **multifocal**, seeding remote regions of the bladder. Bladder cancer frequently has **occult micrometastases** and generally metastasizes to lymph nodes, viscera, and bones.

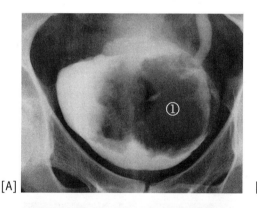

[A]

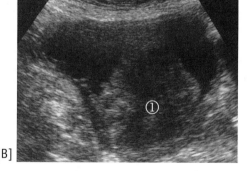

[B]

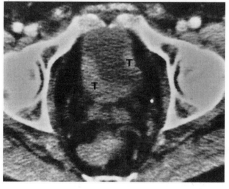

[C]

BLADDER CANCER

High-grade tumors frequently elaborate hCG, which is a marker for an aggressive tumor and signifies an unfavorable prognosis.

Epidemiology Men are affected more commonly than women (2.7 to 1), with those affected usually between the ages of 50 and 70. Risk factors include exposure to industrial solvents and dyes, **cigarette smoking**, chronic *Schistosoma hematobium* infection, and mechanical trauma from stones. With invasive disease, the 5-year survival rate is approximately 50%; with metastatic disease at diagnosis, the mean survival is < 2 years.

Management Treatment depends on the stage of the tumor. Endoscopic resection and periodic follow-up with cystoscopy and biopsy are appropriate for low-grade superficial lesions. Intravesical chemotherapy reduces the risk of recurrence after resection. Invasive disease requires partial or radical cystectomy with lymph node dissection in combination with radiation and/or chemotherapy. The small bowel may be used to create a continent reservoir for urine (KOCH POUCH).

Complications Local recurrences and distant metastases are very common.

Atlas Link ⬛U⬛C⬛V⬛1 PM-P2-053

MINICASE 366: ORCHITIS

Inflammation of the testes
- associated with mumps virus, *Escherichia coli*, and STDs such as *Chlamydia*, *Neisseria gonorrhoeae*, or *Mycobacterium tuberculosis*
- presents with scrotal and testicular swelling and tenderness
- treat with analgesics, ice packs, antibiotics

Atlas Link: ⬛U⬛C⬛V⬛1 PG-M2-082

MINICASE 367: TORSION OF THE APPENDIX TESTIS

Ischemia of a rare embryologic remnant similar to the testicle in the scrotum
- caused by spermatic cord torsion, causing venous outflow obstruction and subsequent arterial occlusion to the testicle
- seen more frequently with cryptorchidism
- presents with sudden-onset scrotal pain
- characteristic blue dot visible within the testicle
- duplex US reveals lack of spermatic artery flow
- treat with emergent detorsion, orchiopexy if the testicle is necrotic

ID/CC   A 61-year-old **black man** complains of increasing **difficulty initiating urination, a slow stream**, and persistent dripping at completion.

HPI   He states that he wakes up **four times per night to urinate** (NOCTURIA) and complains of **intermittent painful urination** (DYSURIA). Yesterday he noticed **blood in his urine** (HEMATURIA). Directed questioning reveals that he started having **back pain** 4 months ago (metastases to spine). The patient also reports **increased urinary frequency**.

PE   VS: normal. PE: abdominal and lung exam normal; tenderness on spinous process of **vertebrae** (bone metastases); testes normal; rectal exam reveals normal sphincter tone and a diffusely enlarged prostate gland (benign hyperplasia) with a **painless, hard, nodular, irregular mass** in posterior lobe.

Labs   CBC: **anemia** (Hb 8.5 gm/dL) (from chronic disease). Slightly elevated BUN and creatinine (due to obstruction of trigonal ureteral entrance to bladder); **elevated acid phosphatase** (also increased in prostatitis, prostatic massage or instrumentation, and extraprostatic disease); **hypercalcemia** (bone metastases); **elevated alkaline phosphatase** (increased in bone metastases); **elevated PSA** (false positives may occur with benign prostatic hypertrophy, instrumentation, and prostatitis).

Imaging   **[A]** CT, pelvis: large prostate (P) with massive left aortoiliac **lymph node** (1); note the bladder (B) and colon (C). **[B]** MR, pelvis: a different case showing prostate carcinoma (1) invading the lower part of the bladder. **[C]** Nuc, bone scan: another case with multiple **diffuse metastatic lesions**, primarily in the **axial skeleton. [D]** MR, spine: a different case with a large thoracic vertebral metastasis.

Pathogenesis   **Endocrine** (hormonal) influences can affect **genetically** predisposed individuals (e.g., blood group A), with **dietary** and **environmental** factors leading to tumor development. Prostate cancer may be symptomatic or may be discovered on routine rectal exam; it is associated with kidney failure (due to ureteral obstruction), bone metastases (pain), and neurologic deficits in the legs. Dissemination occurs first to the base of the bladder and seminal vesicles. Lymphatic spread is to the iliac, periaortic, and sacral lymph nodes; bone metastases are to the axial skeleton, pelvis, and sacrum. **Staging**: A = nonpalpable; B = localized nodule; C = periprostatic spread; D = lymph node/distant metastases.

Epidemiology   In men, prostate cancer is the **most common cancer** (160,000 new cases annually) and is the second leading cause of cancer death, with a high prevalence among older men but low clinical incidence. It is more common among **African Americans** and has a low incidence among Asians. The most common site is the periphery of the posterior lobe; the most common type is **adenocarcinoma**; the most common presenting pattern is stage C. Postvasectomy patients appear to be at increased risk.

Management   The chance of cure increases with **early detection** (rectal exam, PSA, transrectal ultrasound with biopsy). **Diagnose and stage** with perineal/transrectal ultrasound-guided biopsy, plain films of the axial skeleton, technetium scans, and cystoscopy. Local disease is **curable** (via radical prostatectomy); the primary complications of surgery are **incontinence and impotence. Local extension is treated with radiotherapy and metastatic disease with antiandrogen therapy** (orchiectomy, estrogen). Ketoconazole (inhibits adrenal androgen production), leuprolide (an LHRH agonist), and flutamide (a nonsteroidal antiandrogen) are alternative **antiandrogen therapies. PSA** is highly specific for assessing **disease recurrence**.

Complications   Perineal tumor invasion (pain), metastatic disease (bony metastases), obstructive uropathy, and UTIs.

Atlas Links   ⬚⬚⬚⬚⬚ PG-P2-063, PM-P2-063

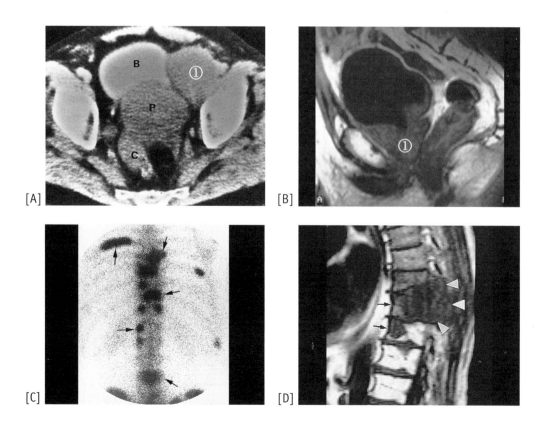

[A]   [B]   [C]   [D]

ID/CC	A 55-year-old **white male** presents with right flank pain and **blood in his urine** without dysuria.
HPI	The patient is an avid **smoker**. He also complains of nausea, headache, **weight loss**, and **fever**.
PE	VS: fever (38.6°C); hypertension (BP 150/96). PE: alert; no jaundice; no cyanosis; lungs clear to auscultation; **palpable, painful mass in right flank**; no costovertebral angle tenderness; **left varicocele.**
Labs	CBC: **Hb 17.4 gm/dL** (due to erythropoietin secreted by tumor; advanced disease may present with anemia); leukocytosis with no left shift. **Elevated ESR; hypercalcemia. LFTs: AST and ALT normal. PT prolonged** (out of proportion to transaminases); **elevated alkaline phosphatase** (bone metastases). UA: **hematuria.**
Imaging	**[A]** IVP: right **pelvicaliceal distortion** by lower pole tumor mass. **[B]** CT (contrast enhanced): **tumor** (1) **with increased vascularity**; incidental simple cyst (2) in the left kidney. **[C]** Angio, renal: a different case with abnormal **tumor neovascularity** in the left upper pole kidney. **[D]** XR, pelvis: another case with metastatic **lytic bone destruction** of the right inferior and superior pubic rami.
Pathogenesis	Renal cell carcinoma accounts for 85% of renal parenchymal cancers and classically presents with **hematuria, flank pain**, and **palpable mass**. Patients frequently present with **painless hematuria** (gross or microscopic), pathologic fracture, skin nodules, or left varicocele (tumor extension to left renal artery). Renal cell carcinoma is associated with **cigarette smoking**, defects in chromosome 3, and radiation (old contrast media). **Multiple** lesions **metastasize to the lungs** ("CANNONBALL" LESIONS), liver, local lymph nodes, adrenals, and long bones. **Paraneoplastic syndromes** are frequently observed, i.e., hypertension (secondary to renin secretion or vascular effects), hypercalcemia, galactorrhea, Cushing's syndrome, Stouffer's syndrome (nonmetastatic hepatic dysfunction), **erythrocytosis** (secondary to elevated erythropoietin levels), and **fever** (secondary to endogenous pyrogen production). CT scan is diagnostic and is the staging procedure of choice.
Epidemiology	Renal cell carcinoma is more common in **whites** and **males**. The most common type is adenocarcinoma from tubular cells. Predisposing factors include **adult-onset polycystic kidney disease, von Hippel–Lindau disease**, tuberous sclerosis, and renal cysts in

hemodialysis patients. Because of earlier diagnosis, 5-year survival is now approximately 70%.

Management Work up with bone and liver scan, CT, and CXR. Early stages with no local spread can be treated with radical nephrectomy (adrenal, local nodes, distal ureter). If solitary, lung metastases may be resected. Treat osseous metastases with radiotherapy. Advanced disease can be treated with medroxyprogesterone, vinblastine, α-interferon, IL-2, and lymphocyte-activated killer cells, although results are not very encouraging. Recurrences may occur even 15 years after primary tumor resection.

Complications Intratumoral bleeding, leg edema, and **varicocele** due to vena cava thrombosis; high-output cardiac failure (AV shunting); pulmonary embolism, renal colic due to clots, polycythemia, metastatic disease (lungs, bone), paraneoplastic syndromes (e.g., hypercalcemia), obstructive uropathy, and **pathologic fractures**.

Atlas Link ⬛ⓊⒸⓋ⓵ PM-P2-064

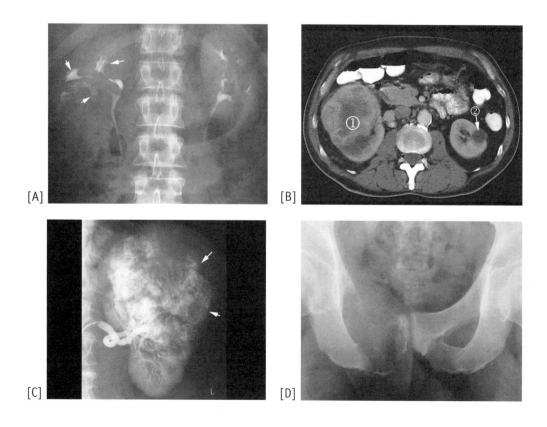

[A] [B] [C] [D]

ID/CC A 28-year-old man presents with a **painless enlargement of his testes** of several months' duration.

HPI The patient was initially unconcerned because the enlargement was painless. He has become more concerned because of continued growth and an increased sensation of heaviness. He reveals that he was diagnosed with **cryptorchidism** in the right testicle as an infant; the condition was corrected by orchiopexy at age 1.

PE VS: normal. PE: in no acute distress; lung and abdominal exams normal; diffuse enlargement of testes noted on GU exam; rectal exam unremarkable.

Labs CBC: **mild anemia. Mildly elevated hCG**; normal α-fetoprotein; **elevated LDH**.

Imaging **[A]** US: intratesticular hypoechoic mass (extratesticular masses are less worrisome). **[B]** MR, testis: well-circumscribed low-intensity right intratesticular mass with normal left testicle. CXR/CT, abdomen and pelvis (to look for metastases): normal.

Pathogenesis Testicular germ-cell tumors are classified as **seminomas** (40% of cases) and **nonseminomas** (embryonal cell carcinomas, teratomas, choriocarcinomas, and mixed-cell types). Non-germ-cell tumors (Leydig cell, Sertoli cell, gonadoblastoma) comprise the remaining 5% to 10%. Seminomas are classified by the M. D. Anderson staging system, in which stage I is confined to the testes, stage II involves retroperitoneal lymph nodes, and stage III involves supradiaphragmatic lymph nodes or viscera. Approximately 5% of patients have a **history of cryptorchidism** (usual histology is seminoma), and 10% have tumors in the contralateral, normally descended testis. Correction with orchiopexy does not decrease

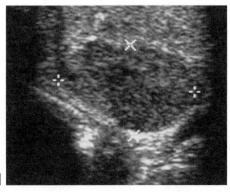

[A]

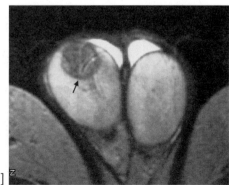

[B]

the risk of future malignancy but facilitates examination. In addition to congenital and developmental factors, exogenous estrogen, trauma, and infections have also been linked with testicular tumors.

Epidemiology Malignant testicular tumors are very rare; the lifetime probability of developing a testicular tumor is 0.2% for a white male. Testicular cancer occurs more frequently on the **right side**, consistent with the predilection of cryptorchidism for the right side.

Management **Inguinal orchiectomy** is required to exclude a tumor or establish the diagnosis. Scrotal approaches and testicular biopsies should not be performed. Postsurgical therapy depends on histopathology and clinical staging as determined by radiologic scanning. Stages I and IIa seminomas (retroperitoneal disease < 10 cm diameter) are treated with radical orchiectomy and **retroperitoneal irradiation alone**, yielding 5-year disease-free survival rates of 98%. High-stage IIb and III seminomas require primary **chemotherapy** (etoposide and cisplatin or etoposide, cisplatin, and bleomycin), yielding complete response in 95% of patients. Surgical resection of residual retroperitoneal masses is appropriate in the presence of masses > 3 cm in diameter, as 40% of these masses harbor residual carcinoma.

Complications Testicular tumors may be complicated by metastases to the retroperitoneum (low back pain), lungs (cough), or vena cava (lower extremity edema), or they may lead to intratesticular hemorrhage. Although 10% of patients are asymptomatic at presentation, another 10% may manifest symptoms of advanced metastatic disease, as most cases are not brought to the physician's attention for 3 to 6 months.

Atlas Links ☐Ⓤ Ⓒ Ⓥ Ⓘ☐ PG-P2-067, PM-P2-067

ID/CC A 21-year-old woman presents with **altered mental status, headache**, right-sided weakness, double vision (DIPLOPIA), and **projectile vomiting**.

HPI She had been drinking with friends 2 hours earlier when she slipped and **hit the left side of her head** on the ground and lost consciousness. She recovered 2 minutes later and was watching TV at home (LUCID INTERVAL) when her symptoms began.

PE VS: no fever (36.7°C); **bradycardia** (HR 40); normal RR (RR 19); **systolic hypertension** (BP 150/70). PE: **confused** and anxious; **disoriented; papilledema**; left pupillary dilatation (MYDRIASIS) and fixation (not reacting to light); deviation of left eyeball outward and downward (left CN III palsy); right-sided weakness and diminished touch and pain sensation; brisk right-sided DTRs; right **extensor plantar response** (BABINSKI'S SIGN); neck supple with no rigidity or pain.

Labs CBC/Lytes: normal. Glucose, BUN, and creatinine normal. UA/ABGs: normal.

Imaging XR, cervical spine (AP and lateral views): no fractures. **[A]** CT, head: **hyperdense convex lens-shaped (lenticular) extra-axial fluid collection (1)** with mass effect and edema. **[B]** A different

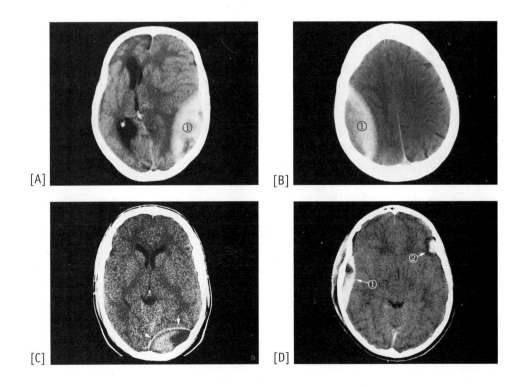

[A] [B] [C] [D]

EPIDURAL HEMATOMA

case with a right parietal epidural hematoma (1). **[C]** Another case with a chronic posterior epidural hematoma. **[D]** Another case with a right temporal epidural hematoma (1) and a "contrecoup" hemorrhage (2) on the left.

Pathogenesis Epidural hematoma is usually caused by rupture of the **middle meningeal artery**; it is usually associated with temporal bone fracture. Less frequently, it may be due to rupture of dural venous sinuses (occipital). **Blood collects between the skull and dura mater**, producing a mass effect. Classically, the patient initially **loses consciousness** and then **regains consciousness and remains asymptomatic** (during which time blood continues to accumulate) **for a variable period of time before neurologic signs appear**; however, only 10% to 15% of patients with an epidural hematoma experience this lucid interval. It is usually associated with **ipsilateral mydriasis** due to CN III palsy **and contralateral hemiparesis**.

Epidemiology Occurs in approximately 1% of patients with head trauma. Any age group may be affected, but those whose work or hobbies predispose to accidents (e.g., skiing) are at higher risk. Delay in recognition leads to a **mortality rate of approximately 40%**.

Management Rising ICP with the potential for herniation makes **early recognition essential** for a successful outcome. Hyperventilate and give IV mannitol. Raise the head of the bed and give antiepileptics as necessary. Treatment is emergent and consists of **surgical evacuation** via **burr holes** and **control of bleeding**.

Complications Complications include cerebral **herniation and death** secondary to raised ICP from the mass effect of the expanding blood (cingulate gyrus herniation under falx, uncal herniation over tentorium, tonsillar herniation through foramen magnum). The mortality rate is as high as 40% to 50% in untreated cases.

Atlas Link ⃞U⃞C⃞V⃞1 PG-P3-010

MINICASE 368: ACOUSTIC NEUROMA

A vestibular nerve schwannoma (if bilateral, suspect neurofibromatosis type 2)
- presents with features of cerebellopontine angle compression and vestibulo-auditory impairment (tinnitus, vertigo, and hearing loss)
- CT/MR show an enhancing cerebellopontine angle mass with an enlarged internal acoustic meatus
- radiation therapy or surgical resection is curative

Atlas Links: ⃞U⃞C⃞V⃞1 PG-A-049, PM-A-049

ID/CC	A 56-year-old **man** presents with **fibrotic bands on both palms** along with **flexion contractures** of the fourth and fifth fingers bilaterally.
HPI	The patient has a history of **alcoholism** and **hepatic cirrhosis**.
PE	VS: normal. PE: localized thickening of palmar fascia bilaterally with palpable longitudinal cordlike bands of tissue on volar aspects of fourth and fifth fingers, drawing both hands into flexion contractures; palmar erythema, bilateral parotid enlargement, and spider nevi (signs of chronic liver disease); icterus; scant pubic and axillary hair; gynecomastia.
Labs	CBC/UA/Lytes: normal. Decreased albumin. LFTs: elevated AST and GGT.
Imaging	XR: no bony abnormalities; MCP and interphalangeal joints normal.
Pathogenesis	The etiology of Dupuytren's contracture is unknown; there may be **genetic susceptibility**. The condition is **often bilateral** and may also involve the feet.
Epidemiology	**More common in men**; seen with increased frequency in patients with **cirrhosis**, in epileptic patients on hydantoin, in diabetics, and in patients status post-MI. It most commonly affects the fourth and fifth fingers. It is also associated with **Peyronie's disease**.
Management	Early cases may be treated with **physical therapy**, night splinting, and gentle stretching. Injection of corticosteroid into the contracture may lead to dissolution. Advanced cases require excision or division of affected fascia. **Surgery** yields good results except when permanent joint changes have occurred in the MCP and PIP joints.
Complications	High rate of recurrence after operative treatment (15% to 20% recurrence).

HAND—DUPUYTREN'S CONTRACTURE

ID/CC	A 40-year-old man presents with **pain, swelling**, and **deformity of the right leg** after a **motor vehicle accident (MVA)**.
HPI	He was thrown forward in the car, and his **knees hit the dashboard**.
PE	PE: right leg **flexed at hip, adducted**, and **internally rotated; shortening** noted; head of femur felt in gluteal region.
Imaging	XR: **femoral head out of acetabulum**.
Pathogenesis	The injury is sustained by trauma directed along the shaft of the femur, with the hip flexed; a severe force is required, as occurs in an MVA. There are three main types of hip dislocations. **Posterior dislocations** are most common and are usually due to a posteriorly directed force on the flexed hip (e.g., knee hitting dashboard). **Anterior dislocations** are rare injuries that are sustained when the leg is forcibly abducted and externally rotated. Clinically, the femoral head is palpable in the groin. In **central fracture dislocation**, the femoral head is drawn through the medial wall of the acetabulum into the pelvic cavity. If skeletal traction fails to reconstitute the acetabular margins, surgical reconstruction of the acetabular floor is necessary.
Epidemiology	Increased incidence in patients who have undergone a total hip replacement or had a posterior wall acetabular fracture.
Management	Reduction of the dislocation under general anesthesia with muscle relaxation, followed by skeletal traction for 6 weeks until the capsule has healed. If a bony fragment is displaced from the posterior acetabular wall, open reduction and internal fixation of the fragment may be required.
Complications	Complications include sciatic nerve damage, recurrent dislocation, and concomitant ligamentous injuries of the knee (e.g., posterior cruciate ligament injury). Joint stiffness and osteoarthritis are inevitable complications.

ID/CC A 65-year-old woman complains of **inability to use and bear weight** on her left leg after tripping on a carpet.

HPI Onset of **menopause** was 20 years ago. She is not receiving hormone replacement therapy or calcium supplements.

PE PE: left leg **externally rotated, shortened, and adducted; tenderness in left groin**; attempted hip movements are painful and associated with severe spasm.

Labs CBC: normal.

Imaging **[A]** XR, left hip: **femoral neck fracture with displacement. [B]** XR, left hip: a different case with an intertrochanteric femoral fracture. **[C]** MR, right hip: another case showing a right femoral neck nondisplaced fracture that was not visible on plain x-ray. **[D]** XR, right hip: another case, status post-right hip pin placement 10 months ago for subcapital fracture, now with avascular necrosis (1) (sclerotic femoral head).

Pathogenesis **Osteoporosis** is an important contributory factor to hip fracture in elderly women, in whom the fracture can result after a

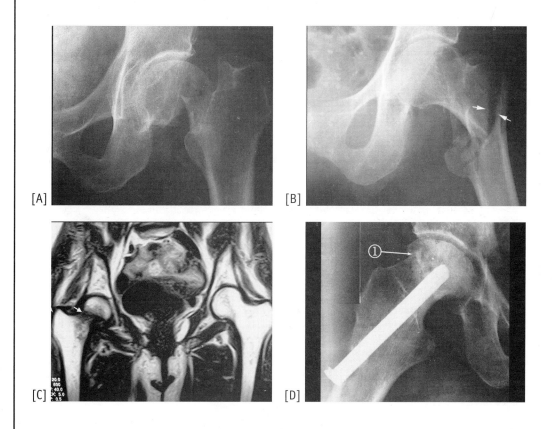

[A] [B] [C] [D]

seemingly trivial fall; in young adults, this fracture is the result of a more severe injury. Fractures are classified as **intracapsular** (subcapital and transcervical) and **extracapsular** (basal and intertrochanteric).

Epidemiology   Most commonly seen in **osteoporotic elderly women**.

Management   **Intracapsular** (subcapital and femoral neck fractures): undisplaced fractures are fixed with screws; displaced fractures require femoral head replacement (hemiarthroplasty vs. primary total hip replacement). **Extracapsular** (basocervical and intertrochanteric hip fractures): a sliding compression hip screw allows the nail to slide along a border that is part of the plate, allowing the fracture to compact during weight bearing. Treat with warfarin postoperatively for DVT prophylaxis.

Complications   **Avascular necrosis of the femoral head**. The blood supply of the head of the femur comes from three sources: retinacular vessels in the capsule, medullary vessels in the femoral neck, and via the ligamentum teres. The main source is via the retinacular vessels, which may be damaged in intracapsular femoral neck fractures. Thus, for intracapsular hip fractures, the risk of avascular necrosis of the femoral head depends on the amount of displacement at the fracture site. Extracapsular fractures do not involve the hip capsule and damage the blood supply, thus running a lesser risk of avascular necrosis of the femoral neck. Other complications include nonunion or malunion with varus angulation and shortening.

MINICASE 369: EWING'S SARCOMA

Undifferentiated bone sarcoma, most commonly affecting the tibial diaphysis
- occurs in adolescence, more commonly in boys
- presents with pain, swelling of the leg, and mild fever, usually associated with a large soft tissue mass
- biopsy is diagnostic
- karyotype may show translocation of the long arms of chromosomes 11 and 22, x-ray shows "onion skin" appearance
- treat with radiation therapy and surgical resection
- regular follow-up is needed owing to the risk of relapse

ID/CC   A 56-year-old **obese** woman presents with **pain** and **stiffness** of the right knee joint.

HPI   Her **symptoms have gradually increased** over the past few years. She has also noticed **swelling and deformity of the joint** and has difficulty walking.

PE   VS: normal. PE: right knee joint **tender; crepitus** on motion; **firm swelling** (caused by underlying bony proliferations) and **joint effusion**; limited motion at joint; examination of hands reveals bony swellings on DIP (HEBERDEN'S NODES) and PIP (BOUCHARD'S NODES) joints.

Labs   CBC: WBC count normal. ESR normal; examination of synovial fluid shows **no evidence of inflammation**.

Imaging   [A] XR, right knee: **narrowing of joint space** (1) (especially on the medial weight-bearing aspect of the joint); subchondral bone **sclerosis** (2); subchondral **cysts** and **osteophytes. [B]** XR, spine (lateral): another case demonstrating a similar degenerative process in the cervical spine with straightening and decreased joint space. **[C]** MR, spine: a different case with severe

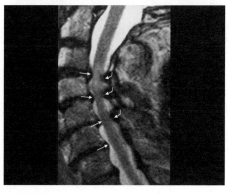

[A]

[B]

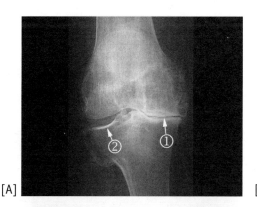

[C]

OSTEOARTHRITIS

cervical spondylosis; the thecal sac is indented by multiple disk protrusions and osteophytes.

Pathogenesis   Osteoarthritis is associated with increased water content in the articular cartilage and loss of articular cartilage. The mechanism may be related to alterations of the collagen network that allow for the absorption of excessive amounts of water and for the subsequent **loss of proteoglycans**, thus altering the mechanical properties of cartilage. The articular cartilage cannot be replaced or repaired, perhaps because the normal pattern of the collagen fiber network cannot be regenerated by chondrocytes.

Epidemiology   The most common of the rheumatic diseases; incidence **increases with age**. Osteoarthritis occurs with **equal frequency in men and women**, but different patterns of joint involvement predominate; osteoarthritis of the hands and knees is more common in women, whereas that of the hips is more common in men.

Management   Conservative treatment includes **analgesia** with NSAIDs, **weight loss**, and **physiotherapy**. Exercise regimens have been shown to lessen pain. Assistive devices such as a walker or cane can help unload excessive forces on the knee. Intra-articular corticosteroid injections may also control inflammation and thus provide relief of symptoms. In patients with severe pain and significant limitation in activities of daily living that have not responded to conservative measures, **replacement arthroplasty** (total knee replacement) provides significant relief and mobility.

Complications   Complications of osteoarthritis include persistent pain and stiffness, resulting in interference in activities of daily living.

Atlas Links   ☐☐☐☐ **SUR-044**   ☐☐☐☐ PG-P3-073

MINICASE 370: FOREARM—GALEAZZI'S FRACTURE

Fracture of the radial shaft and concomitant dislocation of the distal radioulnar joint
- presents with arm pain following trauma
- x-ray of both the wrist and the forearm is required to evaluate fracture
- treat with closed reduction of the dislocation (accomplished by supination of the forearm), open reduction and internal fixation of the fracture

ID/CC	A **19-year-old male** college student complains of **pain** in the right knee and lower thigh and mild **swelling** of the joint that began 3 days after he played football.
HPI	Otherwise healthy, he has been having **dull, aching pain** for several weeks that **worsens at night**. The pain is not relieved with aspirin (rule out osteoid osteoma). He denies any malaise, fever, chills, diaphoresis, headache, nausea, vomiting, or weight loss.
PE	VS: normal. PE: no acute distress; no jaundice; lower thigh and knee are slightly **swollen, tender**, and **warm** with **limitation of movement** by contracture; no inguinal lymphadenopathy.
Labs	Elevated **alkaline phosphatase**. LFTs: normal. Immunoelectrophoresis normal (rules out multiple myeloma); calcium, phosphorus, and PTH normal; biopsy reveals **osteogenic sarcoma**.
Imaging	**[A]** XR, knee (lateral): permeative **osteolytic metaphyseal** lesion in the distal end of the femur; cortical involvement with **"sunburst"** appearance. **[B]** XR, knee (PA): a different case with spiculated periosteal reaction and **dense sclerosis** (1). **[C]** XR, tibia: another case with lifted **periosteal new bone** in a triangular shape (CODMAN'S TRIANGLE).
Pathogenesis	Osteogenic sarcoma, also called **osteosarcoma**, is a primary malignant tumor of bone that occurs most frequently in patients with **retinoblastoma gene mutations** and in those who have undergone **radiation**. It affects the **ends of long bones** in the following order of frequency: **distal femur, proximal tibia, proximal humerus, and pelvis**. The prognosis is better for tumors in the tibia than for those in the femur. Patients may present with a **painless mass** or with **dull, aching pain following a minor injury**. Articular cartilage provides a barrier to tumor spread. The tumor metastasizes most frequently to the lungs.
Epidemiology	The **most common primary malignant tumor of bone**; usually affects **younger individuals** (teens) and shows a **male predominance**. **Paget's disease of bone** is a predisposing factor, accounting for the second peak of incidence in middle age. **Chronic osteomyelitis** is also a predisposing factor.
Management	**Aggressive resection** (wide surgical resection with reconstruction versus amputation) with **radiation therapy** and **chemotherapy**. A possible primary tumor with bone metastases should be sought.

OSTEOGENIC SARCOMA

Radiotherapy is much more successful in **Ewing's** than in osteosarcoma (and is used mainly for patients who refuse amputation).

Complications **Pathologic fracture** and **secondary infection; metastatic disease** (lung metastases) and **lymphatic involvement**.

Atlas Link UCV1 PM-P3-074

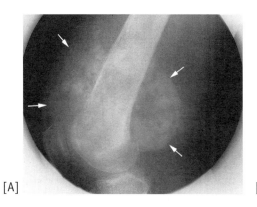 [A]

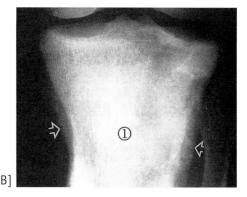 [B]

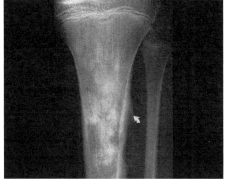 [C]

ID/CC	A **10-year-old boy** presents with **pain in the right lower shin, malaise, and fever** of 3 days' duration.
HPI	Two weeks ago, he fell and **injured** his right shin. There is no family history of sickle cell disease.
PE	VS: **fever** (38.5°C). PE: **redness, swelling**, and **tenderness** over right lower tibia; movements limited by pain; patellar tap demonstrated over knee joint (sympathetic effusion).
Labs	CBC: **leukocytosis** (16,500) with predominant **neutrophilia**. ESR elevated (68 mm/hr). Blood culture yields *Staphylococcus aureus*; bone aspiration reveals frank pus.
Imaging	**[A]** XR, right tibia: normal initially. **[B]** Nuc (technetium-99): **increased uptake** at the proximal tibia in the metaphyseal area (positive before changes appear on x-ray). **[C]** XR, right tibia: periosteal **new-bone formation** (periosteal reaction) at the upper tibial metaphysis (earliest sign to appear on x-ray; takes about 7 to 10 days). **[D]** XR, tibia: a different case showing chronic osteomyelitis with extensive sclerosis.
Pathogenesis	*S. aureus* is the most common organism responsible for osteomyelitis. In patients with sickle cell disease, *Salmonella* osteomyelitis is common. The organisms reach the bone via the **hematogenous route**. Suppuration occurs, leading to **bone necrosis**; pus forms under the periosteum, strips it and penetrates through, forming a sinus. Necrotic bone is called **sequestrum**; the new subperiosteal bone that forms around the dead bone, forming a shell, is called **involucrum**. The **lower femoral metaphysis** is the most common site involved; other sites include the upper end of the tibia as well as the humerus, ulna, radius, and vertebral bodies.
Epidemiology	Acute osteomyelitis is usually a **disease of childhood** and is more common among **boys**, probably because boys are more prone to injury; **immune-compromised individuals and diabetic adults** are also susceptible.
Management	**Penicillinase-resistant antibiotics** in combination with an **aminoglycoside** for at least **6 weeks**; resolution of fever and decreasing ESR are good indicators of the effectiveness of such therapy. **If pus has formed at the site of osteomyelitis, it must be operatively drained.**
Complications	Complications of acute osteomyelitis include chronic osteomyelitis, acute pyogenic arthritis (in joints where the

metaphysis is intra-articular), pathologic fracture (bone may be weakened by infection or surgical intervention) and growth plate disturbances, and dissolution of the femoral head with subsequent limb-length inequality.

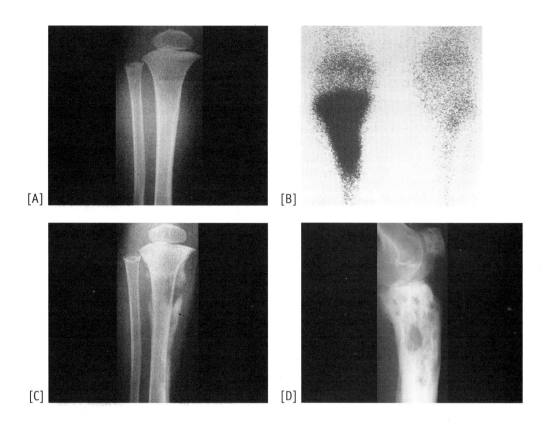

[A]

[B]

[C]

[D]

ID/CC A 23-year-old student presents with right shoulder pain after **falling backward and sideways onto his outstretched hand** (forced abduction and external rotation); he cannot move his right arm.

HPI He noticed **deformity** of his shoulder and had to **hold his right arm**.

PE VS: normal. PE: a **depression** is easily palpable under the acromion; humeral head palpable through axilla; normal sensation over deltoid and active firing of deltoid (no evidence of axillary nerve palsy).

Labs CBC: normal.

Imaging [A] XR, shoulder (AP): **humeral head dislocated anteriorly** and displaced to the **subcoracoid** position with a **greater tuberosity fracture (1)**.

Pathogenesis The glenohumeral joint is the most frequently dislocated joint owing to its poor stability (the glenoid cavity is small in relation

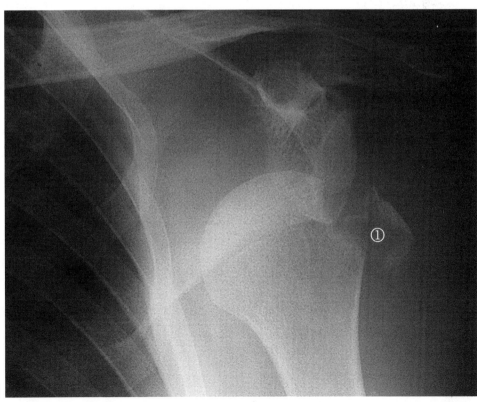

[A]

to the humeral head); injuries usually result from a fall on the arm in forced abduction and external rotation but can also result from a direct fall on the posterolateral shoulder. The **contour of the shoulder** characteristically appears **square** (loss of normal rounded shape). The humeral head and glenoid cavity may fracture, and injury to the brachial plexus may lead to an **axillary nerve palsy** (leading to **inability to abduct** the arm due to deltoid paralysis and **hypesthesia** on the lateral shoulder skin). Associated **rotator cuff tears** also occur on occasion. In a posterior dislocation the anterior shoulder looks flat, the coracoid process is prominent, and the patient cannot externally rotate his arm.

Epidemiology **Greater than 85% of all shoulder dislocations are anterior** (the humeral head lies in front of the coracoid process of the scapula); capsular tears predispose patients to recurrent dislocations. Posterior dislocations are less common, and inferior dislocations are rare. **Seizures** may lead to anterior or posterior dislocations.

Management **Rule out nerve damage and fractures** via AP, lateral, and axillary x-ray views. Success is inversely proportional to the time that has elapsed between injury and reduction. One method of closed reduction involves tying a weight onto the patient's arm for 10 minutes with the patient lying prone and the affected arm hanging over the table; when the muscles relax, the dislocation reduces. **Cooper's method** (HIPPOCRATIC METHOD) involves pulling the extended arm with the patient supine while using the bare foot in the axilla as a fulcrum. **Kocher's method** involves applying traction on the humerus with the elbow at 90 degrees, **externally rotating** the arm, maintaining traction, and then **adducting** the arm and **internally rotating** it until a click is heard. **X-ray confirmation is required after reduction**. In young patients, **immobilize** for 3 weeks; in the elderly, begin range-of-motion exercises earlier to prevent stiff shoulder. Analgesics are usually sufficient for pain control, but sedation or general anesthesia may be needed for reduction. **Recurrent dislocations** require soft tissue/capsular surgical repair.

Complications Recurrent dislocation, rotator cuff tear, lateral tear, glenoid fracture, axillary nerve injury, and brachial plexus dysfunction.

SHOULDER DISLOCATION

ID/CC A 40-year-old man complains of **acute-onset severe back pain** that began while he was **lifting a heavy object**.

HPI The pain worsens with movement, coughing, and straining and **radiates to the right buttock and thigh**. He also complains of patchy **sensation loss** in the left leg. The patient denies having any history of urinary or bowel incontinence.

PE Back pain with associated tenderness to palpation and paraspinous muscle spasm; normal anal sphincter tone; no evidence of sciatica with straight leg raising; 2+ symmetric Achilles and patellar DTRs with downgoing toes bilaterally; no evidence of any motor defects in lower extremities bilaterally.

Imaging XR, lumbar spine: **loss of lumbar lordosis** and **vertebral osteophytes**; no evidence of fracture. **[A]** and **[B]** MR, spine: left posterolateral **disk herniation** at L5–S1, **producing nerve root compression**. The right S1 nerve root is clearly seen.

Pathogenesis Degenerative changes of the annulus fibrosus and paraspinal ligaments may lead to herniation of the disk substance (nucleus pulposus) into the spinal canal; minor trauma is usually sufficient to precipitate symptoms. The herniation of disk material may compress one or more nerve roots, leading to **radicular pain** and to either **sensory or motor deficits**. The risk of nerve root compression is greater if the spinal canal is congenitally narrow or has become narrow as a result of hypertrophic changes in the facet joints. **Lumbar disk herniation most commonly affects the S1 nerve root at the L5–S1 level or the L5 nerve root** at the L4–L5 level, although extrusion of a large disk fragment may compress more than one root.

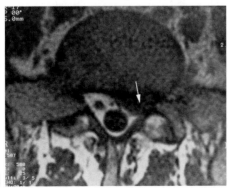
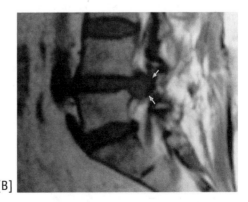

Epidemiology	Degenerative disk disease most commonly occurs in **smokers** and those exposed to **vibrational stress**. Also, patients who repeatedly **lift heavy objects** are at increased risk for back injury.
Management	Conservative treatment includes **complete bed rest, analgesia, traction, and mobilization in a corset. Surgical treatment** is indicated when there is bladder or bowel paralysis, muscle weakness, or failure of conservative therapy; operative therapy includes surgical removal of the disk following laminectomy or chemonucleolysis (disk is dissolved with chymopapain).
Complications	Motor weakness, sensory loss, cauda equina syndrome, back spasms, persistent pain and instability.

MINICASE 371: FOREARM—MONTEGGIA'S FRACTURE

A fracture of the upper third of the ulna with dislocation of the radial head caused by a fall on an outstretched hand
- presents with inability to pronate and supinate the forearm
- x-ray shows fracture with dislocation
- treat by open reduction and internal fixation of the ulna followed by cast immobilization

---

MINICASE 372: HIP—SLIPPED CAPITAL FEMORAL EPIPHYSIS

The most common deformity occurring in adolescence
- the proximal femoral metaphysis externally rotates and displaces anteriorly from the capital femoral epiphysis
- presents with an antalgic gait and severe hip or knee pain
- x-ray shows displacement or widened epiphyseal plate
- treat by fixation of the epiphysis to the metaphysis with a cannulated screw

ID/CC A 50-year-old woman presents with pain, swelling, and deformity of the left wrist.

HPI One hour ago, she **fell on her outstretched left hand**.

PE VS: normal. PE: tenderness and irregularity of lower end of radius with characteristic **"dinner fork" deformity**; radial styloid process palpated at level of ulnar styloid process (normally it is situated higher than the radial styloid); supination of distal fragment; no pain on passive extension of fingers (rule out compartment syndrome); palpable radial and ulnar pulses.

Imaging **[A]** XR, wrist (PA): disruption of bony trabeculae and **cortical stepoff** in an extra-articular Colles' fracture. **[B]** XR, wrist (PA): a different case with an intra-articular comminuted fracture. **[C]** XR, wrist (lateral): the distal articular surface of the radius faces dorsally (dorsal tilt is the most characteristic displacement).

Pathogenesis Colles' fracture almost always results from **a fall on an outstretched hand**. The fracture line runs transversely just proximal

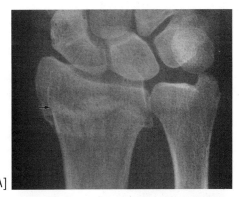

[A]   [B]

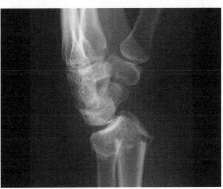

[C]

to the distal articular surface. Displacements (dorsally and radially), impaction of fragments, tilt, and supination can occur.

Epidemiology   While it is the **most common fracture in individuals older than 40 years**, it is also very common in children and is frequently seen with rollerblading, trampoline, and bicycle injuries.

Management   Treat via **closed reduction and splinting** followed by **above-elbow casting** after swelling resolves. Indications for operative treatment include Galeazzi fractures (radius fractures with associated dislocation of the ulna at the distal radioulnar joint), intra-articular comminuted fractures, failure to obtain an adequate bony alignment with closed reduction, neurovascular entrapment, and soft tissue interposition at the fracture site.

Complications   Complications include stiffness and edema of the hand, malunion with angulation, associated pain from subluxation of the distal radioulnar joint, median nerve compression symptoms, tendon rupture, Sudeck's atrophy (reflex sympathetic dystrophy), and compartment syndrome.

MINICASE 373: PAGET'S DISEASE OF BONE

Osteoclastic destruction of bone, initially with excessive osteoblastic repair, producing sclerosis, seen in late adulthood
- presents with pain, sensorineural hearing loss, increase in hat size, and tibial bowing
- markedly elevated alkaline phosphatase and increased urinary excretion of hydroxyproline
- treat mild disease with NSAIDs, severe disease with calcitonin or bisphosphonates
- complications include high-output CHF, pathologic fractures, and osteosarcoma

---

MINICASE 374: PELVIC FRACTURE

Usually as a result of high-energy trauma, with multiple associated injuries that take precedence unless there is fracture-related hemorrhage
- presents with pain, pelvic instability, hypotension, and signs of visceral injury (hematuria, rectal bleeding, or neurovascular deficits of the lower extremities)
- labs may reveal low hematocrit
- pelvic imaging (XR-AP, inlet/outlet tilt, and pelvic CT) to demonstrate the fracture, evaluate accompanying visceral damage (urethrogram, cystogram, and arteriography)
- treat with external fixation followed by internal fixation after hemorrhage is controlled
- complications include injury to pelvic organs and hemorrhage/shock

MINICASE 375: REFLEX SYMPATHETIC DYSTROPHY

Sympathetic pain that may be idiopathic or secondary to fractures, sprains, or trivial soft tissue injury
- presents with intense, burning pain, edema, and thin, shiny skin
- radiograph of the involved extremity may reveal severe osteopenia
- treat with tricyclic antidepressants or gabapentin, TENS, or neural blockade
- complications include lifelong, debilitating pain

MINICASE 376: SPINE—PROLAPSED INTERVERTEBRAL DISK

A common cause of low back pain
- the disk prolapses through the annulus fibrosus and compresses the nerve root
- presents with low back pain, pain shooting down the leg (SCIATICA), loss of DTRs, and leg paresis
- MR demonstrates disk herniation
- treat with bed rest, NSAIDs, surgery only for refractory radiculopathy or myelopathy

MINICASE 377: SPINE—SPONDYLOLISTHESIS

One vertebra slips forward relative to the one below, usually L5 or S1, owing to a breach in ossification between the lamina posteriorly and the body anteriorly
- presents with chronic backache and a palpable "step" in the line of spinous processes
- spine x-ray shows "Scottie dog" defect in pars interarticularis vertebrae
- consider spinal fusion for severe cases

MINICASE 378: WRIST—BARTON'S FRACTURE

A distal intra-articular radial fracture with dislocation of the radiocarpal joints
- presents with wrist and hand pain after trauma
- x-ray reveals the fracture and dislocation
- treat with open reduction and internal fixation to restore the anatomic alignment of the articular surface

MINICASE 379: WRIST—SCAPHOID FRACTURE

Fracture typically caused by a fall on an outstretched hand
- presents with tenderness in anatomical snuff box
- on x-ray, fracture line may be inapparent for 2 weeks after fall, consider MRI
- treat by immobilizing the wrist in knuckle-to-elbow plaster, including the thumb as far as the interphalangeal joint
- complications include avascular necrosis of the proximal segment, delayed union, nonunion, and future osteoarthritis of the joint

ID/CC A 71-year-old man presents with **shortness of breath** (DYSPNEA) **on exertion** and cough that have worsened over the past 6 months.

HPI He states that he has noticed progressive **weakness, weight loss**, and loss of appetite. Yesterday he **coughed up blood** (HEMOPTYSIS). He has smoked since age 17 and currently **smokes three packs a day**. He has a chronic productive cough (most common presenting symptom) and also complains of an embarrassing **increase in the size of his breasts** (GYNECOMASTIA) as well as **wrist pain**.

PE VS: no fever (36.9°C); tachypnea (RR 21). PE: no acute distress; barrel-shaped chest (underlying emphysema); lungs with scattered **crackles bilaterally**; wheezing and **diminished breath sounds** in upper right lung field; **grade IV clubbing of fingers** bilaterally with tenderness on wrist percussion (HYPERTROPIC PULMONARY OSTEOARTHROPATHY); **acanthosis nigricans** (paraneoplastic syndrome) on both lower legs; purpuric spots on chest and arms.

Labs CBC: anemia (Hb 8.0 gm/dL); moderate leukocytosis; **thrombocytosis**; eosinophilia. Increased ESR. Lytes/LFTs: normal. Hypercalcemia; bronchial washings and cytology of sputum reveal **large-cell carcinoma**.

Imaging [A] CXR: **peripheral mass** (1) in the right apex with hilar lymph node metastasis (2). [B] CT, chest: a different case showing a smaller peripheral spiculated mass. [C] MR: another case with a right apical mass invading the mediastinum. XR, long bones: **osteolytic metastases** in the spine and left humerus. XR, wrist: **periosteal elevation** (due to hypertrophic pulmonary osteoarthropathy).

Pathogenesis Lung cancer can arise as a result of a variety of caustic environmental agents, most notably **cigarette smoking**. Other causes include radon gas, arsenic, ionizing radiation, mustard gas, heavy metals (nickel and chromium, which also cause nasal cavity cancer), asbestos (mesothelioma), and industrial ether (small cell cancer). Types include adenocarcinoma, squamous cell (EPIDERMOID; most benign), small cell (OAT CELL; most virulent), and large cell. **Adenocarcinoma** is generally peripheral and leads to distant metastases, also causing nonbacterial verrucous (MARANTIC) endocarditis, hypertrophic pulmonary osteoarthropathy, and thrombophlebitis. **Bronchoalveolar** (a subtype of adenocarcinoma)

LUNG CARCINOMA

metastasizes late, is bilateral, and is associated with copious watery or mucoid sputum. **Squamous cell** cancers begin centrally (intraluminal bronchial growth, diagnosed with cytology), metastasizes late to regional lymph nodes, and may cause Pancoast's syndrome, hypercalcemia (due to ectopic PTH-like peptide secretion), and hypertrophic pulmonary osteoarthropathy; 10% cavitate. **Small cell** cancer is also central, narrows bronchi by extrinsic compression, metastasizes early to lymph nodes, and causes Cushing's syndrome (ectopic ACTH), SIADH (excessive ADH), myasthenia (EATON–LAMBERT SYNDROME), and serotonin secretion. **Large cell** is usually peripheral and produces distant metastases, increased gonadotropins, and gynecomastia. All types may cause anemia, dermatomyositis, acanthosis nigricans, thrombocytosis, and eosinophilia.

Epidemiology Although lung cancer is **the second most common cancer in both men** (after prostate cancer) **and women** (after breast cancer), it accounts for the **most cancer deaths in both genders**. Additionally, a sharp increase in incidence has recently been seen in women. Overall, the **5-year survival rate is approximately 10%** but varies widely with type and stage.

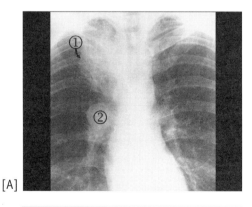

[A]

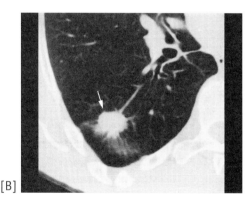

[B]

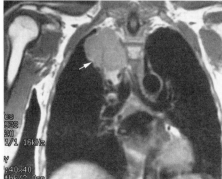

[C]

Management   First-line therapy for small-cell cancer is multiagent chemotherapy and thoracic radiotherapy. Prophylactic cranial irradiation (to decrease the risk of CNS metastasis in patients in remission) may play a role. Non-small-cell cancers confined to regional lymph nodes and one hemithorax may be surgically resected. Sufficient lung tissue must remain after surgery to permit adequate gas exchange. More advanced tumors may benefit from chemotherapy and radiation. **Inoperable** tumors include those with distant metastasis or esophageal, contralateral lymph node, pericardial, tracheal, or superior vena caval involvement. Palliative therapy generally involves radiation and may involve surgery or endobronchial laser resection.

Complications   Advanced disease commonly leads to **superior vena cava syndrome** (neck, arm, and face swelling and arm pain due to compression of the superior vena cava), **hoarseness** (due to recurrent laryngeal nerve paralysis), and **Pancoast's syndrome** (apical invasion of the cervical sympathetic plexus and arterial and venous trunks, causing muscle wasting, arm pain, reduced pulse, engorgement of the jugular vein, and Horner's syndrome [ptosis, miosis, anhidrosis, and enophthalmos]). Other complications include metastatic disease, paraneoplastic syndromes (e.g., SIADH), and airway obstruction.

Atlas Links   ⬚U⬚C⬚V⬚1   PG-P2-085, PM-P2-085

MINICASE 380: PSEUDOGOUT

Joint inflammation due to calcium pyrophosphate dihydrate (CPPD) crystal deposition
- most often affects the knee
- synovial fluid shows rhomboid-shaped, positively birefringent crystals
- treat with colchicine and NSAIDs

Atlas Link: ⬚U⬚C⬚V⬚1 PM-P3-090

ID/CC	A 13-year-old girl on **mechanical ventilation** in the ICU develops acute **respiratory distress, right pleuritic chest pain** referred to the right shoulder, and bluish coloration of the fingers and tongue (CYANOSIS).
HPI	She was **intubated** in the ER two days ago following a house fire in which she sustained smoke inhalation injury (with burning of the upper respiratory tract).
PE	VS: mild fever (38.3°C); **tachycardia** (HR 125); **hypotension** (BP 80/40); tachypnea. PE: **cyanotic** (late manifestation) and in acute respiratory distress; **tracheal deviation** to the left; poor chest expansion on inspiration, with **hyperresonance** on right (TYMPANITIC); **absence of breath sounds in right lung field; decreased tactile fremitus** in right hemithorax; marked **JVD**; regular rate and rhythm; S$_1$ and S$_2$ normal; PMI shifted to left.
Labs	CBC: leukocytosis. Lytes/UA: normal. ABGs: **decreased P$_{O_2}$** (HYPOXEMIA) and **increased P$_{CO_2}$** (HYPERCAPNIA).
Imaging	**[A]** CXR: **hyperlucency** of the right thorax and **mediastinal shift** to the left. **[B]** CXR: a different case with left tension pneumothorax demonstrated by hyperlucency, a collapsed and **retracted lung**, and an **inverted** left **hemidiaphragm**.
Pathogenesis	In a tension pneumothorax, a **one-way valve is established**, permitting air to flow into the pleural space during inspiration without allowing efflux during expiration. Thoracic pressure rises, leading to collapse of the ipsilateral lung, mediastinal shift and tracheal deviation to the contralateral side, and severely diminished venous return and contralateral ventilation.

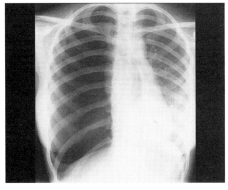

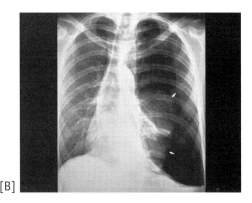

[A]   [B]

Epidemiology **Trauma** and **high-pressure ventilatory support** cause the vast majority of tension pneumothoraces.

Management **Presumptive diagnosis should be based on clinical suspicion**; do not wait for x-rays to treat. Life-saving decompression with a **large-bore needle** converts a tension pneumothorax to an open one (associated with less hemodynamic compromise). Insert the needle just above the rib edge (avoiding the neurovascular bundle beneath the rib) in the second intercostal space 2 cm lateral to the sternum (in children) or in the midclavicular line (in adults). A **chest tube** should then be placed in the fifth intercostal space, midaxillary line, and directed superiorly.

Complications Unrecognized tension pneumothorax is associated with respiratory failure, hemodynamic compromise (secondary to decreased venous return), and death. Long-term sequelae are rare after successful treatment.

PULMONARY

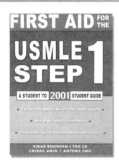
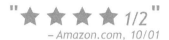
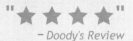
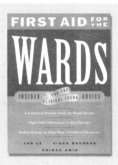
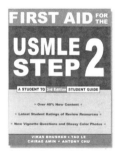
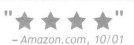
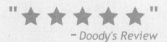
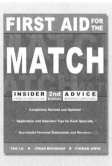